Dental Public Health
A PRIMER

Dental Public Health

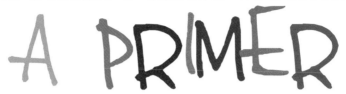

Meera Patel
BDS (Lond)   MFGDP RCS
General Dental Practitioner, Leicester

Nakul Patel
BSc (Hons)   MB BS (Lond)
Pre-Registration House Officer, Barts and The London

Forewords

Kevin Lewis
Dental Director, Dental Protection

Raman Bedi
Eighth Chief Dental Officer for England

Illustration and Design

Gaman Patel
Freelance Artist and Printer

Nakul Patel
Freelance Artist

Radcliffe Publishing
Oxford • Seattle

Radcliffe Publishing Ltd
18 Marcham Road
Abingdon
Oxon OX14 1AA
United Kingdom

www.radcliffe-oxford.com
Electronic catalogue and worldwide online ordering facility.

British Library Cataloguing in Publication Data

A catalogue record for this book is available from the British Library.

ISBN-10: 1 85775 647 9
ISBN-13: 978 1 85775 647 0

Typeset: Gaman Patel and Nakul Patel
Illustration and Design: Gaman Patel and Nakul Patel
Printed and Bound: Alden Press (Malaysia)

CONTENTS

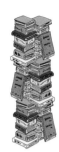

Chapter 1: Concepts of Dental Public Health   1

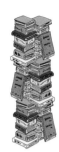

Chapter 2: Epidemiology in Dentistry   7

Chapter 3: Health Promotion   21

CONTENTS

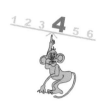
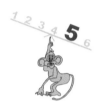

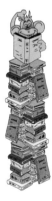

FOREWORD

For different reasons, undergraduate dental students and general dental practitioners tend to be preoccupied with the 'small picture'. But in reality, every 'small picture' is simply one part of a much bigger picture, and this refreshing book conveniently provides both.

Dental public health can seem a long way removed from the immediacy of the filling you are placing this afternoon, and let's face it - not everyone is turned on by epidemiology and healthcare economics. That is precisely why I think that readers will be surprised and quickly engaged by this book. The unusual presentation and delivery of the information is a metaphor for the challenge that the writers have perceptively identified and taken on - that of taking large amounts of potentially intimidating and complex information, and making it simple, accessible and easy to understand. Unless you can get the dental public health message off the library shelf and into the thinking of the undergraduate, you will always struggle to get it from the graduate to the point of delivery.

It may be no coincidence that my own passion for preventive dentistry was born and nurtured during my undergraduate days at The London Hospital (later to become part of Barts and The London, Queen Mary's School of Medicine and Dentistry), from where Meera and Nakul Patel both graduated. My path also crossed with that of Ray Croucher (one of the contributors to this book) over 25 years ago when I had my own preventive-based general practice in Peterborough, and he was actively involved in the Dental Health Study at the University of Cambridge. Indeed, I recall that he even filmed a much younger Kevin Lewis, talking to children in the preventive unit of my Peterborough practice. Serendipity indeed.

Prevention and health promotion makes as much sense now as it did then, although UK dentists face different challenges when trying to make it a practical reality today. Inevitably, at a time of unprecedented change in UK dentistry, the text of this book has been overtaken here and there by legislative and regulatory reforms, but the central message remains undiminished.

Dental public health may be 'big picture' in one sense, but it becomes 'small picture' whenever patients come into contact with dental health professionals. That is why I would hope that this innovative foray into making the subject interesting, meaningful, relevant and memorable for undergraduate dental students, will reach a much wider audience than that.

As the twin concepts of skill mix and teamworking become the norm in general and specialist practice, there is a new and large batallion of potential dental health educators and health promoters who will not have seen the inside of a dental school or school of dental hygiene and therapy. All the more reason to hope, therefore, that the message of this book reaches them.

A genuine desire to make a difference, infectious enthusiasm, and the desire to communicate, are all important tools for healthcare professionals to possess. In the field of prevention and health promotion they are critical. It is clear that in Meera and Nakul Patel, the torch continues to burn brightly which augers well for the future.

Kevin Lewis
Dental Director, Dental Protection
Associate Editor, 'Dental Practice'
Formerly General Dental Practitioner

FOREWORD

This is a remarkable book which will not replace many of the standard textbooks in Dental Public Health but will complement them.

When I observe my 16-year-old son studying he, like many of his contemporaries, leaves his text books unopened, uses the internet, and discusses subjects with friends via MSN and mobile phones; a new generation learning new information and using tools that were not available to many of us when we were undergraduates.

Meera Patel has just recently graduated from dental school and, with her brother Nakul, have shown they understand the mindset of this new generation of students. They have taken the undergraduate dental public health curriculum and asked two questions, what does the final year student need to know and how can we make it fun to learn? To this end they have been very successful in producing a highly amusing and informative book. They have put a degree of energy back into a subject that is all too often presented in a dull and uninteresting manner.

This book will appeal to all members of the dental team, especially when they are revising for their exams. The standard textbooks will still be needed to better understand the subject, but I can imagine that many future undergraduates will be thankful for this revision guide.

Raman Bedi

Professor Bedi was the eighth Chief Dental Officer for England (2002-2005). He implemented some of the most significant improvements in dentistry since the creation of the National Health Service, addressed oral health inequalities, established infection control standards and published and oversaw the implementation of the 2004 Dental Workforce Review. In 2005 he led the global declaration on the future of child oral health, and in 2006 became the Director of the Global Child Dental Health Taskforce.

PREFACE

Why Write About Dental Public Health?

Most dental students dread revising dental public health (DPH) as they find it tedious and mind-numbing. Nevertheless, the subject is full of fascinating concepts and ideas that may appear a bore over reams of picture-less pages lined with microscopic black text. In retaliation, we have transformed the subject matter into an easily digestible pictorial format that develops and maintains the interest of the reader.

The naive first-year dental student may perceive the subject as irrelevant, however, it is only later that they come to appreciate the implications of public health issues and concepts such as 'prevention rather than cure'. As Downer (1994) described, DPH is the science and art of preventing oral disease, promoting oral health and improving the quality of life through the organised efforts of society.

As the book title suggests, this is an introductory textbook and certainly not a definitive guide to the subject. It does however cover all the major aspects that would be expected of an undergraduate dental course. This textbook should be supplemented with course notes and additional core textbooks should more detailed explanation be needed. Although primarily targeted at undergraduate dental students it can be used by general dental practitioners, lecturers and other allied health professionals as a quick cross-reference guide or for teaching.

The book can be used at home, university, in the clinic or even on the bus or train. It can be used as a revision guide for examinations. It can be used as a beginner's guide to DPH issues for the relative novice.

This book is very simple to follow and understand, covering the core concepts of DPH. We have incorporated mnemonics and acronyms. Also ideas and theories have been illustrated with lots of colourful pictures. This will help students retain what they learn for the rest of their lives! We aim to make what is perceived to be a boring dental subject, fun to learn!

The Book Structure

The book is divided into three main sections:

- **Core Text:** The first part includes five chapters which make up the bulk of the book. Each of these chapters begins with the aims and objectives of the chapter. The pages in these sections are generally divided into two, the left side consists of text and the right is pictographical representation of the text. Many pictures, graphics, colours, mnemonics and acronyms have been used to make learning both effortless and enjoyable. The chapters conclude with likely exam questions, including short-answer questions (SAQ), long-answer questions (LAQ) and essay questions which will enable the reader to test their knowledge. The sixth chapter is a useful glossary of terms which frequently come up in exams.

- **Passing The Exams:** The second section describes the functioning of the brain, how best to revise and tips on examination technique.

- **Additional Sources of Information:** The final section contains a list of websites, sources of epidemiological data, further reading material and references.

How Best To Use The Book

We suggest that you have a quick scan of the 'Passing The Exams' section first. Understanding the basic functioning of the brain will assist your revision by making it more effective. Now you are ready to attack each of the chapters. Start by reading the aims and objectives, then the notes, making use of the revision tips you have learnt. Highlight salient points, add post-it notes, scribble over the margins, deface the book if you must... but make each page memorable! You can now cross-reference with your lecture notes and read additional material from core texts if certain topics need more detail. Finally, try out the exam questions to test your knowledge.

We hope you enjoy your journey with us...

We welcome any comments about the book.   **Meera Patel and Nakul Patel**

Chapter 2: Epidemiology In Dentistry

INTRODUCTION

Determinants of Health Diagram

Adapted and reproduced from: Dahlgren G and Whitehead M. (1993). *Tackling social inequalities in health: what can we learn from what has been tried?* Technical Background Paper for International Seminar on Tackling Inequalities in Health. Ditchley Park, Oxford. London, King's Fund.

Chapter 3: Health Promotion

DETERMINANTS OF HEALTH (2)

Determinants of Health Diagram

Adapted and reproduced from: Dahlgren G and Whitehead M. (1993). *Tackling social inequalities in health: what can we learn from what has been tried?* Technical Background Paper for International Seminar on Tackling Inequalities in Health. Ditchley Park, Oxford. London, King's Fund.

THE CONCEPT OF HEALTH PROMOTION

Common Risk Factor Approach Diagram

Adapted and reproduced from: Sheiham A and Watt RG. (2000). The common risk factor approach: a rational basis for promoting oral health. *Community Dentistry and Oral Epidemiology.* 28:399-406.

Health Promotion Logo

Adapted and reproduced from: WHO. (1986). *The Ottawa Charter for Health Promotion.* Geneva, World Health Organization.

Chapter 4: Oral Health Care

BARRIERS TO ACCESS (4)

Health Promotion Logo

Adapted and reproduced from: WHO. (1986). *The Ottawa Charter for Health Promotion.* Geneva, World Health Organization.

Chapter 5: Preventive Dentistry

PREVENTIVE STRATEGIES: ORAL CANCER (2)

Health Promotion Logo

Adapted and reproduced from: WHO. (1986). *The Ottawa Charter for Health Promotion.* Geneva, World Health Organization.

ABOUT THE AUTHORS

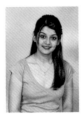

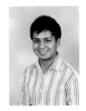

Meera Patel
BDS (Lond)   MFGDP RCS
General Dental Practitioner
Leicester

Nakul Patel
Bsc (Hons)   MB BS (Lond)
Pre-Registration House Officer
Barts and The London

Meera Patel graduated from Barts and The London, Queen Mary's School of Medicine and Dentistry in 2003. She was a high achiever in her year group gaining distinctions in Dental Public Health, Psychological, Ethical and Legal aspects of Dentistry, Adult Oral Health and Child Dental Health.

She also achieved an impressive list of prizes which include Drapers' College Prize, British Society of Restorative Dentistry Prize, Communication Skills Prize, Barts and The London Alumni Association Elective Prize, CWF Thomas Prize, and a membership with the International Association of Student Clinicians (American Dental Association).

Following graduation she did her vocational training in Ilkeston, Derbyshire. She is a member of the BDA Branch Council for the Trent region. She takes pleasure in teaching and has lectured to vocational trainers, vocational dental practitioners and dental students across the country.

At present she is working as a General Dental Practitioner in Leicester, where she is developing her interest in orthodontics, implantology and dental health education.

Nakul Patel graduated in Medicine from Barts and The London, Queen Mary's School of Medicine and Dentistry in 2005. He also achieved a First Class Honours BSc degree in Experimental Pathology, from which he learnt many of his research skills.

His prizes include John Blandy Prize, Barts and The London Alumni Association Elective Prize, The Vandervell Foundation Prize, Convocation Trust Prize, Altounyan Prize in Therapeutics, Barts and The London Association Honours Colours, Student Staff Committee Colours and Badminton Club Colours.

He is currently working as a pre-registration house officer (foundation year one) in London. Since his admission to medical school, he has been keen to be involved in medical education. He represented the student body in the student-staff committee and soon became student chair of that group. Here he helped with teething problems in the new medical curriculum.

He is currently co-authoring another illustrated textbook for medical students.

They are strong believers in effective time management and through this book they would like to make public health issues effortless and enjoyable to learn. They hope that this book will capture the enthusiasm for the subject that they share.

ABOUT THE CONTRIBUTORS

Professor Raymond Croucher
Professor of Community Oral Health

A graduate of the London School of Economics he completed graduate studies in Canada before returning to the UK where he held research posts at the University of Cambridge and University College London. He was appointed Senior Lecturer in Dental Public Health at Barts and The London, Queen Mary's School of Medicine and Dentistry in 1989 and was awarded a personal chair in Community Oral Health in 2001. His current post is Deputy Director (Research) in the Institute of Dentistry and Senior Tutor for Dental Postgraduate Taught Courses. In addition he represents Queen Mary's University of London on the Management Group for the Health Foundation's Consortium for Healthcare Research.

His research career has focused on psycho-social risk factors for oral diseases. Initially he worked in dental health education, developing and implementing innovative school-based programmes such as 'Natural Nashers'. A current interest has been upon stress as a risk factor for periodontal disease and the role of tobacco use in oral diseases. This latter interest stems from his role as Manager of a Tobacco Cessation Programme for the Bangladeshi community of East London, in which tobacco chewing by women is prevalent. He is concerned to develop collaborative primary care activity and evidence-based public policy to combat tobacco use - both smoked and chewed.

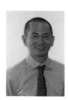

Dr Allan Pau
Clinical Senior Lecturer in Dental Public Health

Allan Pau is Senior Lecturer in Dental Public Health at Barts and The London, Queen Mary's School of Medicine and Dentistry. Following his undergraduate dental education, he worked as a general dental practitioner and a community dental officer before returning to postgraduate studies. In his current post, he is involved in dental public health teaching at undergraduate and postgraduate levels, as well as clinical supervision of undergraduates. His research interests include the epidemiology of dental pain and dental education.

Professor Wagner Marcenes
Professor in Oral Epidemiology

Professor Marcenes completed his PhD in Epidemiology and Public Health at University College London in 1991, and was immediately appointed Lecturer at University College London School of Medicine and at Barts and The London, Queen Mary's School of Medicine and Dentistry. He was promoted to Senior Lecturer in 1999 and in 2002 he was the first in the UK to be appointed as Professor of Oral Epidemiology. Currently, he is the Senior Dental Postgraduate Tutor, and the leading lecturer in Oral Epidemiology, Basic Statistics and Evidence-Based Dentistry. He is currently Director of the Behavioral Science and Health Services Research group of the International Association of Dental Research; serves as a member of the editorial board of Community Dentistry, Oral Epidemiology and Oral Health and Preventive Dentistry.

Professor Marcenes is prominent internationally in the field of social epidemiology pertaining to oral conditions. His seminal work on the psychosocial determinants of oral health behaviour and disease significantly contributed to the understanding of the social causation of oral diseases. He has also conducted several epidemiological oral health surveys among children and adults at a local, national and international level.

Centre for Adult Oral Health
Institute of Dentistry
Bart's and The London Queen Mary's School of Medicine and Dentistry
Turner Street, Whitechapel, London E1 2AD

ACKNOWLEDGEMENTS

It has been a long yet interesting journey and many people have assisted us along the way. We would like to acknowledge all those who have helped us reach our destination with their kind assistance, suggestions, criticisms and continuing support.

Ms Gillian Nineham for giving us this wonderful opportunity along with the entire team at Radcliffe Publishing, who gave their whole-hearted assistance

Barts and The London, Queen Mary's School of Medicine and Dentistry for giving us an excellent foundation on which to build our medical and dental careers

Leicester City Football Club for the use of their club logo

Dr Ana Beatriz Oliveira Gamboa for liaising with the tutors at Barts and The Royal London

Ms Lisa Harris at the Dental Defence Union for assistance with the roadside dentistry section

Professor Parveen Kumar, who has been a source of inspiration throughout our careers

Dr Kapil Patel for his ongoing faith in us to complete our journey

And above all our mother, Sangita Patel, for her endless cups of tea and hot meals!

ABBREVIATIONS

A&E	Accident and Emergency
BDS	Bachelor of Dental Surgery
BPE	Basic Periodontal Examination
BSc	Bachelor of Science
CAL	Clinical Attachment Loss
CDO	Chief Dental Officer
CDS	Community Dental Service
CPD	Continuing Professional Development
CPITN	Community Periodontal Index of Treatment Need
CRFA	Common Risk Factor Approach
DMF	Decayed, Missing, Filled (Index)
dmfs	Decayed, Missing, Filled Surfaces (deciduous teeth)
DMFS	Decayed, Missing, Filled Surfaces (permanent teeth)
dmft	Decayed, Missing, Filled Teeth (deciduous teeth)
DMFT	Decayed, Missing, Filled Teeth (permanent teeth)
DOH	Department of Health
DPB	Dental Practice Board
DPH	Dental Public Health
GDC	General Dental Council
GDP	General Dental Practice
GDS	General Dental Service
GPT	General Professional Training
HDS	Hospital Dental Service
ICT	Information and Communication Technology
LLL	Life Long Learning
MBBS	Bachelor of Medicine and Bachelor of Surgery
NHS	National Health Service
NICE	National Institute for Health and Clinical Excellence
NRT	Nicotine Replacement Therapy
PCD	Professionals Complementary to Dentistry
PCT	Primary Care Trust
PDS	Personal Dental Services
RCS	Royal College of Surgeons
RCT	Randomised Controlled Trial
RSD	Roadside Dentist
SDP	Salaried Dental Practitioner
SHA	Strategic Health Authorities
SOHI	Subjective Oral Health Indicators
TDI	Traumatic Dental Injuries
VT	Vocational Training
WHO	World Health Organization

DENTAL EDUCATION

Philosophy Of Dental Education

Dental education should aim to provide the student with the following:

- A comprehensive understanding of health and disease and their determinants as they affect individuals and communities.
- An ability to develop a professional practice based on scientific and ethical principles and the effective use of resources.
- A commitment to maximise the well-being of patients and the community as a central value.
- A concern with and responsibility for broader social issues such as equity and justice in health and the social and environmental causes of ill-health.

To achieve the above aims, students should develop the following knowledge, beliefs and competencies:

Clinical: the ability to recognise disease, interpret investigations, formulate diagnoses and treatment plans

Management: as managers of small organisations, the ability to organise, co-ordinate and lead the dental team

Political Advocacy: the ability to help groups and communities recognise their own health needs and organise to achieve them

Ethical: an understanding of the principles of ethical conduct and the ability to apply them appropriately in the context of dental practice

Inter-Personal: the ability to understand and communicate with patients, influence their behaviour through communication and education and form relationships with patients which enhance therapeutic outcomes

Scientific: an understanding of scientific principles and the ability to apply them in dental practice. The ability to evaluate knowledge concerning the causes of disease and the benefits derived from the technologies used to treat oral disease

Technical: the ability to employ those technical procedures necessary to treat oral disease

Dental Public Health Undergraduate Curriculum

The dental public health curriculum for undergraduates is summarised below:

- Appreciate the different dimensions of health and measures of oral health status
- Recognise the profession's wider responsibilities towards the community as a whole
- Recognise evidence-based approaches to management and be able to make appropriate judgements
- Epidemiological knowledge of common dental illnesses including dental caries, periodontal diseases, oral cancers and traumatic dental injuries
- Ability to interpret basic statistical and epidemiological data
- Understand that health promotion involves helping individuals and communities to benefit from increased control over their own health with the intention of improving it
- Appreciate the sociological aspects of health care, including the reasons for the widely varying oral and dental needs of different sections and age groups within the population
- Recognise social, cultural and environmental factors which contribute to health or illness and the capacity of health care professionals to influence these
- Awareness of economic and practical constraints affecting the provision of healthcare
- Appreciate the complexity of dental service delivery including the different methods of payment and employment of dentists and the role of different professional groups
- Appreciate the need for inter-professional collaboration in prevention, diagnosis, treatment and management of disease
- Awareness of equity of service provision and barriers to access including for those with special needs
- Understand the principles of clinical governance
- Understand the principles of health promotion and apply them when in contact with patients, especially with regards to tooth brushing with fluoridated toothpastes, diet and nutrition, tobacco avoidance and public health measures such as fluoridation
- Be familiar with the practice of preventive care including oral health education and oral health promotion
- Awareness of the successes and limitations of preventive dentistry and the potential for further progress

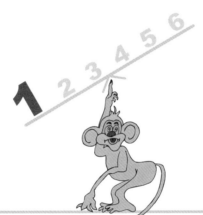

Concepts of Dental Public Health

CHAPTER 1

1

AIMS AND OBJECTIVES

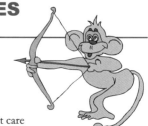

Introduction

Aim

To understand the general concepts of dental public health

Objectives
- Define dental public health
- Describe the activities between public health practice and individual patient care

What Are Health And Oral Health?

Aims
- Recognise that health professionals and lay people have different concepts of health
- Recognise that subjective oral health indicators are developed to supplement clinical measures

Objectives
- Describe the concept of health for health professionals, WHO and the general public
- Identify different dimensions of health
- Define the term 'subjective oral health indicators'
- Describe the properties of 'subjective oral health indicators'
- Describe the use of 'subjective oral health indicators' in oral health research

INTRODUCTION

Definition

Dental Public Health (DPH) is defined as the science and art of preventing oral disease, promoting oral health and improving the quality of life through the organised efforts of society (Downer *et al.,* 1994).

DPH issues can be targeted at different levels:
- Dental or oral
- Individual or population
- Oral or general health

DPH is concerned with making diagnoses, establishing the cause and effects of the disease, and finally implementing appropriate interventions.

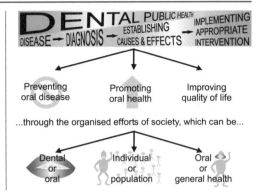

Criteria For Selection Of Dental Public Health Solution

A public health problem is determined if the following criteria are met:
- Feasible to apply **Knowledge** across the population
- **Resources** can be made available
- The condition has a major **Impact** upon the society or individual
- The condition is **Serious** and widespread and in the population
- Ability to **Prevent**, cure or alleviate the condition

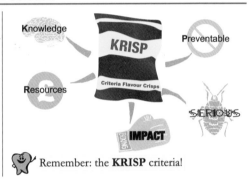

Remember: the **KRISP** criteria!

Core Functions Of Public Health

The three core functions of public health are assessment, policy development and assurance (Turnock *et al.,* 1994). **Assessment** involves reviewing the community's health needs by investigation of adverse events and current health measures. This is followed by analysing the determinants of health and supply of resources. **Policy Development** entails the formation of social support networks and good communication systems (e.g. between the public, health authorities and the media). The local needs are then prioritised, after which an action plan can be developed. **Assurance** involves carrying out and evaluating the action plan. A final important stage involves informing and educating the public about positive health behaviours.

Functions

ASSESSMENT
- Assess health needs of community
- Investigate adverse events and health measures
- Analyse determinants of disease and existing resources

POLICY DEVELOPMENT
- Advocacy
- Prioritising needs
- Planning for the community

ASSURANCE
- Implementation and evaluation of mandated programmes
- Informing and educating the public

Individual Patient Care And Public Health Practice

The table illustrates the stages of activity involved in both individual and public health:

Stages of activity	Individual health	Public health
Data collection	History and Examination	Survey/ observations
Problem identification	Diagnosis	Data analysis
Identifying solutions	Treatment plan	Programme plan
Seeking approval	Informed consent	Approval by health authority
Action	Treatment	Implement programme
Meeting costs	Forms of payment (NHS vs Private)	Types of finance
Evaluation	Treatment goals	Programme goals

 Remember: 'Dental Protection IS A Must Everytime!'

WHAT IS HEALTH?

Definitions

Concepts of *health* are perceived differently by individuals. **Health professionals** define health as freedom from a medico-dental defined disease, where *disease* is defined as abnormalities in anatomical structures or physiological or biochemical process. In 1948, the **World Health Organization** (WHO) defined health as a state of complete physical, social and mental well-being, and not merely the absence of disease or infirmity (Nutbeam, 1998). The positive and negative attributes of this definition:

Positive	Negative
Positive statement	Unrealistic & idealistic
Emphasis on well-being	Static rather than adaptive
Multi-dimensional	Who defines what health is?

Lay person's concept of *illness* is the subjective interpretation of problems perceived to be health related (i.e. 'How do I feel?').

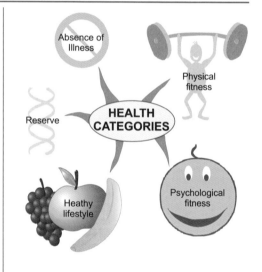

Health And Lifestyle Survey

The health and lifestyle survey by Blaxter (1990) highlighted six key categories of health. These are:
- Absence of illness (no aches and pains)
- Ability to function (unrestricted in work and play)
- Leading a healthy lifestyle (eating healthily)
- Physical fitness (high energy and vitality)
- Psychological fitness (happy and relaxed)
- As a reserve (having good genes)

Other factors that influence people's ideas of health include age, class, gender and race. **Age and Gender:** The concept of health for a young man is physical strength, for a young woman it is energy, vitality and being able to cope, whereas for a middle-aged person it is mental well-being and contentment. **Ethnic Groups:** Asians conceptualise health as being able to function; in contrast, Afro-Caribbeans believe health to be energy and physical strength.

These variations help the health professional:
- Appreciate the gap between need and demand
- More effective communication with patients
- Make health promotion and education more successful
- Understand the 'informal' health care system

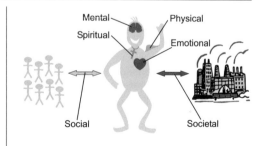

The continuum between health and disease

HEALTH ⬌ DISEASE

Dimensions Of Health

Health can be described by a number of interrelated factors. These may affect people to differing degrees during one's life (Ewles and Simnett, 1999).
- **Physical Health:** Body functioning properly
- **Mental Health:** Thinking clearly and coherently
- **Emotional Health:** Recognising emotions
- **Social Health:** Making and maintaining relationships
- **Spiritual Health:** Behaving ethically
- **Societal Health:** Linking health to the environment

WHAT IS ORAL HEALTH?

Definitions

Oral health is defined as a standard of health of the oral and related tissues which enables an individual to eat, speak or socialise without active disease, discomfort or embarrassment and which contributes to general well-being.

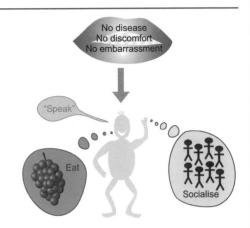

Measures Of Oral Health Status

Measuring health becomes difficult as ideas vary widely and are subjective. The DMF Index and Periodontal Index are examples of two measures of oral health status. They measure past disease and contribute little to the understanding of the oral cavity or subjective symptoms (refer to Chapter 2).

Subjective Oral Health Indicators

Subjective Oral Health Indicators (SOHI) are measures of the extent to which dental and oral disorders disrupt normal social functioning and bring about major changes in behaviour. They measure (Locker, 1988):

- **Discomfort and Pain:** Self-reported and not directly observable symptoms
- **Disease:** Pathological process
- **Impairment:** Disease leading to anatomical loss, structural abnormality, disturbance in biochemical/physiological process
- **Functional Limitation:** Restrictions in normal body functioning
- **Disability:** Limitation to perform activities of daily living
- **Handicap:** Inability to conform to expectations of groups to which they belong (i.e. unable to eat foods of choice, reduced eating pleasure, deterred from eating with others)

SOHI can be used in treatment planning and policy decisions. They:

- Recognise that oral diseases are social and behavioural in origin
- Provide better predictors of need as current clinical measures are of limited validity
- Fulfil government's need for planning and evaluating data

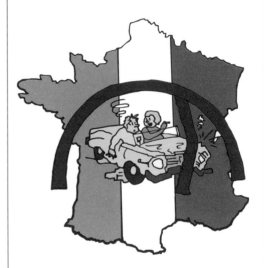

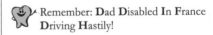
Remember: **D**ad **D**isabled **I**n **F**rance **D**riving **H**astily!

Example Of SOHI Study

The table below shows an example of how SOHI are used in oral health research (Newton *et al.,* 2003):

Study	The self-assessed oral health status of individuals from White, Indian, Chinese and Black Caribbean communities in South-East England
Who	Cross-sectional survey of 336 individuals drawn from the 4 ethnic groups
Measures	SOHI
Findings	Significant differences between ethnic groups on all but one of the SOHI scales. Age and ethnicity (especially Chinese) predict the reporting of self-assessed oral symptoms and the impact of these symptoms

QUESTIONS

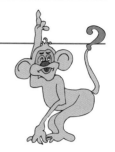

Short Answer Questions

1. Define dental public health. (1 mark)
2. List the core functions of public health. (3 marks)
3. List the positive and negative aspects of the WHO definition of health. (2 marks)
4. What are the advantages of Subjective Oral Health Indicators (SOHI) in treatment planning and policy decisions? (2 marks)

Long Answer Questions

Write short notes on the following topics. Up to 4 marks will be awarded for your answer.
1. How is a public health problem determined?
2. List the stages of activity for individual patient care and public health practice.
3. List and describe the Subjective Oral Health Indicators (SOHI). Illustrate your answer with an example.

Essay Question

You will be awarded up to 20 marks for your answer.
1. Health is defined differently by different people. Discuss the concepts of health, illness and disease, including the dimensions of health.

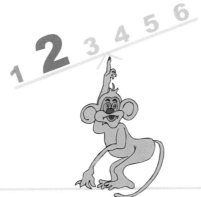

Epidemiology in Dentistry

CHAPTER 2

2

AIMS AND OBJECTIVES

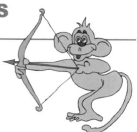

Introduction

Aim

To introduce the concept of epidemiology

Objectives

- Define epidemiology
- Understand the difference between statistical and causal association
- Understand the stages of epidemiological reasoning

Research Design, Critical Appraisal and Evidence-Based Dentistry

Aim

To explore the role and importance of evidence-based activity for the provision of good quality oral health care

Objectives

- Define longitudinal and cross-sectional studies
- Distinguish between prospective and retrospective studies
- Define and compare observational and interventional studies
- Understand and assess the difference between descriptive and analytical epidemiology

Systematic Review And Meta-Analyses

Aim

To understand the importance of systematic reviews and meta-analyses

Objectives

- Understand the difference between systematic reviews and traditional reviews
- Explain why meta-analyses are used

Epidemiology Of Dental Caries

Aim

To understand the trends of dental caries in the UK and their implications in delivering oral health care

Objectives

- Define dental caries
- List the WHO criteria for the diagnosis of dental caries
- Explain the criteria for assessing an index
- Be aware of the shortcomings of the DMF index
- Describe the general trends and prevalence of dental caries over the past few decades
- Discuss factors associated with caries decline

Epidemiology Of Periodontal Disease

Aim

To understand the trends of periodontal disease in the UK and their implications in delivering oral health care

Objectives

- Understand the basis for the definition of periodontal disease
- Be aware of the shortcomings of the periodontal indices
- Describe the trends in periodontal disease in the UK
- List the individuals at risk from periodontal disease

Epidemiology Of Traumatic Dental Injuries

Aim

To understand the trends of traumatic dental injuries (TDI) in the UK and their implications in delivering oral health care

Objectives

- Describe the trends in dentoalveolar trauma in the UK
- List the causes of TDI
- List the factors considered if you suspect a non-accidental injury

INTRODUCTION

Definition

Epidemiology is the study of the distribution of disease or physiological condition in human populations and of the factors affecting their distribution. It is important to understand that epidemiology is concerned with the study of populations (i.e. groups of people) not the individual.

Epidemiology is concerned with studying populations (groups of people, not individuals)

Key Principles

Epidemiology is concerned with the frequency and distribution of disease, and the determinants of health.

- **Frequency of disease:** Involves measurement of disease and quantification of existence or occurrence of the disease.
- **Distribution of disease:** This is related to time, place and people. *Time:* Whether the disease is increasing or decreasing over time? *Place:* Where the disease is occurring? *People:* Who is getting the disease within a population?
- **Determinants of health:** Considers whether the characteristics of individuals with a particular disease differ from those without the disease (see Chapter 3 for details).

The prime objective of epidemiology is to judge whether an association between exposure and disease is in fact causal. Human disease does not occur at random therefore there are causal and preventive factors involved.

- **Statistical association:** This refers to the statistical dependence between two variables. It is important to understand that this does not imply cause-effect relationship.
- **Causal association:** Causal association is one in which a change in exposure results in a change in the outcome.

Frequency of disease

Distribution of disease

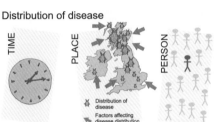

Determinants of health

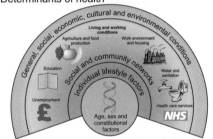

Diagram adapted from Dahlgren and Whitehead, 1993. Adapted and reproduced with permission (see Permissions).

Statistical Association   Causal Association

CAUSE ≠ EFFECT   CAUSE = EFFECT

Epidemiological Reasoning

Epidemiology allows exposure-disease relationship in humans to be measured, and offers possibility of altering the risk through intervention. The following stages are required for epidemiological reasoning:

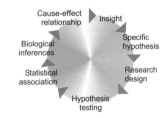

Uses Of Epidemiology

There are many uses of epidemiology.

| Assess **H**ealth care needs, beliefs and behaviour | Explain the **V**ariation in disease | Investigate **C**ausal mechanisms | Investigate possibilities for **P**reventive action | Evaluate the **E**ffectiveness of health services |

 Remember: **H**umans **V**ary **C**onsiderably therefore **P**eople study **E**pidemiology

RESEARCH DESIGN

Definitions

Longitudinal and Cross-sectional Studies: Longitudinal studies are those which investigate changes over time (i.e. individuals are observed more than once). Whereas cross-sectional studies consist of assessing the status of a group of individuals with respect to the presence or absence of both exposure and disease at the same point in time (i.e. like a snapshot in time).

Prospective and Retrospective Studies: Prospective studies are those in which data are collected forwards in time from the start of the study. Whereas retrospective studies are those in which data refer to past events and may be acquired from existing sources.

Observational and Interventional Studies: Observational studies are those in which the researcher collects information on the attributes or measurements of interest but does not influence events. In contrast, interventional studies are those in which the researcher deliberately influences events and investigates the effects of the intervention.

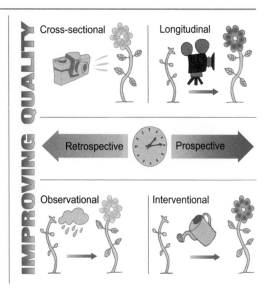

Descriptive And Analytical Epidemiology

Epidemiological research can broadly be divided into descriptive and analytical. *Descriptive epidemiology* is concerned with the distribution of disease, including consideration of which populations or subgroups do or do not develop a disease, in what geographic location a disease is most or least common, and how the frequency of occurrence varies over time. Health professionals can allocate resources efficiently, plan effective prevention and education programmes with the use of descriptive epidemiology. *Analytical epidemiology* focuses on the determinants of disease, with the ultimate goal of judging whether a particular exposure causes or prevents a specific disease. Hypothesis formulated from descriptive studies can be tested by analytical epidemiology.

Descriptive Epidemiology

Observational
- *Case Report:* Consists of a detailed report by one or more clinicians of the profile of a single patient.
- *Case Series:* Consists of a detailed report by one or more clinicians of the profile of a group of patients.
- *Populational Studies (or Ecological or Correlational Studies):* Compare disease frequencies between different populations during the same time period or in the same population at different points in time.
- *Cross-Sectional Study:* Assesses the status of a group of individuals with respect to the presence or absence of both exposure and disease at the same point in time.

Analytical Epidemiology

Observational
- *Case-Control Study:* Consists of selecting a group of individuals who have a disease or outcome being studied and a control group (group of individuals without the disease or outcome being studied), and comparing the proportion of individuals exposed to the factor of interest in each group.
- *Cohort Study:* Consists of classifying individuals on the basis of the presence or absence of exposure to a particular factor, and then following them for a specified period of time to determine the development of disease in each group.

Interventional
- *Randomised Controlled Trial (RCT):* A study in which participants are randomly allocated to intervention or control groups and followed-up over time to assess any differences in outcome rates. RCTs are now well-accepted as the preferred means of evaluating clinical treatments, preventive-screening manoeuvres, and health and educational interventions. Randomisation with concealment of allocation (e.g. use of computer system or table of random numbers to conceal allocation avoids selection bias because it ensures that on average both known and unknown determinants of outcome (prognostic factors) are evenly distributed between groups.
- *Quasi-Randomised Controlled Trial:* A study in which the allocation of participants to intervention or control groups is controlled by the investigator but the method of allocation falls short of genuine randomisation and allocation concealment (i.e. the allocation procedure is entirely transparent before assignment (e.g. allocation by date of birth, hospital record number)).
- *Non-Randomised Trial:* The investigator has control over the allocation of participants to groups, but does not attempt randomisation or quasi-randomisation (e.g. patient or physician preference, patient characteristics and clinical history). The intention here is still experimental rather than observational.

- *Therapeutic Trials:* These are conducted among patients with a particular disease to determine the ability of an agent or procedure to diminish symptoms, prevent recurrence, prevent progression, or decrease risk of death (tooth loss) from that disease.
- *Preventive Trials:* These involve the evaluation of whether or not an agent or procedure reduces the risk of developing disease among those free from that condition at enrolment.

CRITICAL APPRAISAL AND EVIDENCE-BASED DENTISTRY

'One of the most important skills a physician should have is the ability to critically analyse original contribution to the medical literature.'

Albert, 1981

Evidence-based dentistry is a relatively recent approach that will allow you to critically read and assess the quality of such papers and reports, and to understand how to translate the results into your practice. Once qualified, you will be responsible for keeping abreast of new developments in the aetiology, detection, prevention and treatment of dental disorders, including techniques and new materials. This is most effectively achieved through research papers published in scientific journals, in particular systematic reviews, and reports from professional bodies.

This would be fine if all published papers were scientifically sound but, regrettably, the standard of research leaves much to be desired from the statistical point of view. Examples of substandard design and incorrect analysis can be seen in almost any issue of any journal.'

Altman, 1991

Overall Assessment Of Dental Literature

Both descriptive and analytical studies can be assessed by answering the following four questions:

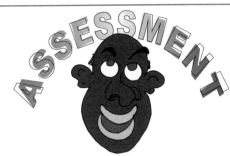

- Will the results help locally? (**Help**)
- Was it ethical to conduct the study? (**Ethical**)
- Was the paper written in a clear, simple and logical way? (**Apparent**)
- Were the findings acceptable taking into account the study design and statistical analysis? (**Design**)

The overall assessment can bring to the surface major and minor problems of the study. Major problems are those concerned with methodology and statistical analysis. Minor problems include the title, abstract, introduction and language used.

Remember: Use your **HEAD** when assessing literature!

Specific Assessment Of Descriptive And Analytical Epidemiology

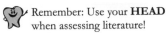

Descriptive Epidemiology

Methodology: Sample Selection and Size
- Was the sample of subjects appropriate with regard to the population to which the findings will be referred?
- Was the source of subjects clearly described?
- Was the method of selection of subjects clearly described?
- Were the criteria for entry into the study (inclusion/exclusion criteria) clearly described?
- Was the calculation of the size of the sample based on pre-study considerations of statistical power?

Methodology: Data Collection
- Were the criteria for outcome measures described or referenced?
- Did the study use sound criteria for outcome measures?
- Were all important outcomes considered?
- Is the number of examiners used in the fieldwork presented?
- Was the examiner(s) trained into the criteria for outcome measures adopted (training and calibration exercise)?

Methodology: Overall Assessment
- Was the study design acceptable?
- Was the study design appropriate to the objective of the study?

Data Analysis
- Were the statistical methods used appropriate for the data?
- Were they used correctly?
- Was sufficient analysis carried out?

Results Presentation
- Is the presentation of statistical material satisfactory?
  - Tables, graphical, numerical
- Was the response rate acceptable?
- Were the validity and reliability of the data collected acceptable?
  - Clinical and non-clinical data
- Are the confidence intervals given for the results? And were they acceptable?

Findings
- Are the findings drawn from the study related to the aim and objectives?
- Are the findings justified taking into account the study design and statistical analysis?

Analytical Epidemiology

Methodology
- Was the assignment of subjects to groups randomised?
- Was the method of creating the randomisation described?
  - Tables of random numbers
  - Computer-generated randomisation
- Were all the subjects who entered the trial properly accounted for at its conclusion?
  - What was the proportion of subjects who completed treatment?
  - What was the proportion of subjects who were followed-up?
  - Were subjects analysed in the groups to which they were randomised?
- Were subjects and study personnel 'blind' to treatment?
  - Double-blind design
  - Single-blind design
  - Not a blind design
- Were the groups similar at the start and end of the trial?
  - Demographic variables (age, sex, social class)
  - Health status
  - Risk factors
- Aside from the experimental intervention, were the groups treated equally?
  - Equal instructions
  - Use of a placebo treatment or a positive control
- Was the post-treatment follow-up long enough to account for the occurrence of the outcome of interest?
  - Latency of outcome
  - Postulated effect of the factor being tested

Results
- How large was the treatment effect?
  - Clinical significance
- How precise was the estimate of the treatment effect?
  - Statistical significance (95% confidence interval)

Unfortunately, not all papers will achieve a 'yes' answer to all the questions in our check list. One should keep in mind that the questions are not equally important. Aspects of presentation, while not unimportant, are clearly less important than fundamental aspects of methodology. Thus, for an overall assessment one should be most concerned about possible bias in the design of the study. One should also be concerned about the data analysis and whether the conclusions were justified. Ethical issues must be addressed. If these points were unacceptable for some reason, the paper is unacceptable.

SYSTEMATIC REVIEW AND META-ANALYSES

Introduction

The basis of systematic reviews is the process of systematically locating, appraising and synthesising evidence from scientific studies in order to obtain a reliable overview of the evidence. An objective and transparent approach is used. Evidence-based health care requires that reliable research evidence is made widely accessible and easily interpretable by those making decisions. Most dentists do not have the time or skill to effectively identify and appraise relevant research.

HIERARCHY OF RESEARCH

Randomised controlled trial
Controlled trial with pseudo-randomisation
Controlled trial with no randomisation
Cohort study
Case control study
Before and after studies
Descriptive studies
(cross-sectional surveys,
case series and
case reports)

A Comparison Of Systematic And Traditional Reviews

The rigorous approach in systematic reviews is in direct contrast to the selective and subjective approach largely used in narrative reviews.

Feature	Systematic Review	Narrative Review
Question	Clear and focused	Often general or broad in scope
Search	Strive to locate all relevant published and unpublished studies to limit impact of publication and other biases	Not usually specified and potentially biased
Selection	Explicit description of inclusion criteria	Not usually specified
Appraisal	Examine systematically the methods used in primary studies and investigate potential biases in those studies	Often do not consider differences in study methods or quality
Data Extraction	Duplicate data extraction in pre-tested forms Strive to obtain relevant published and unpublished data	Often not an objective and reproducible process
Synthesis	Systematic qualitative and quantitative summary	Often unsystematic qualitative

Steps In A Systematic Review

Structured question → Comprehensive data search → Study selection and data abstraction (inclusion criteria and data collection forms) → Quality assessment of studies included → Synthesis of data (results of each study are calculated and often combined statistically, if appropriate) → Interpretation of results and summary of key findings

Meta-analyses

Meta-analyses use statistical methods to combine the results of independent studies and examine the overall trend of results. The statistical combination of results from two or more similar studies is often, but not always, part of a systematic review.

Why use meta-analyses?

- To increase **power**: Individual studies are often not large enough to detect differences in effect
- To improve **precision**: The estimation is more precise when it is based on more information
- To assess formally the factors that may affect **treatment effects**: Allow reasons for differences in results to be investigated

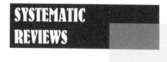

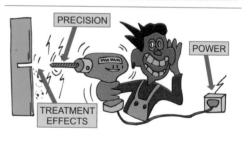

SYSTEMATIC REVIEWS   META-ANALYSES

PRECISION

POWER

TREATMENT EFFECTS

Cochrane Reviews

The Cochrane Collaboration is an international organisation that aims to help people make well-informed decisions about health care. The group prepares, maintains and promotes the accessibility of systematic reviews of the effects of health care interventions. There are 13 Cochrane Centres with around 50 Collaborative Review Groups (including the Oral Health Group), comprising over 9000 individuals from over 80 countries.

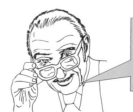

It is surely a great criticism of our profession that we have not organised a critical summary, by speciality or sub-speciality, adapted periodically, of all relevant randomised controlled trials

Archibald Leman Cochrane, CBE FRCP FFCM (1909 - 1988)

EPIDEMIOLOGY OF DENTAL CARIES (1)

Definition

Dental caries is a sugar-dependent infectious disease (Kidd, 1987). The disease affects the calcified tissues of the teeth. It begins with localised dissolution of the inorganic structures of a given tooth surface. This is caused by acids of bacterial origin when fermentable carbohydrates are consumed and leads to disintegration of the organic matrix.

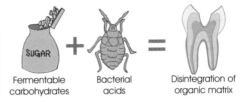

| Fermentable carbohydrates | Bacterial acids | Disintegration of organic matrix |

Clinical Diagnosis

Caries is recorded as present when a lesion in a pit or fissure, or on a smooth tooth surface, has an unmistakable cavity, undermined enamel, or a detectable softened floor or wall.

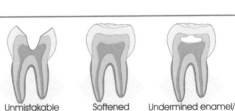

Unmistakable cavity — Softened floor or wall — Undermined enamel/ Hidden cavity

Indices

Dental caries is normally measured using an index. *Index* is defined as a numeric value describing the relative status of a population on a graduated scale with definite upper and lower limits. It is designed to permit and facilitate comparison with other populations classified by the same criteria and methods.

The concept of disease has great implications for the assessment of need for dental care. The broader the scope of the definition of disease, the more healthy people will be included within disease parameters. The narrower the definition of disease, the healthier the population would appear.

The ideal properties of an index are:
- **Validity (sensitivity and specificity)**
- **Quantifiability**
- **Clarity, simplicity and objectivity**
- **Acceptability**
- **Reliability**

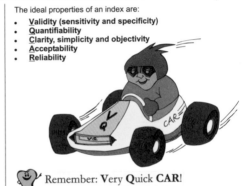

Remember: **V**ery **Q**uick **CAR**!

Measures And Shortcomings

The DMF Index was described in 1937 by Klein and Palmer. It is the most commonly used method of recording dental caries.

- DMFT refers to permanent teeth
- DMFS refers to permanent tooth surfaces
- dmft/dmfs refer to primary dentition

D: Decayed
M: Missing
F: Filled
T: Teeth
S: Surface

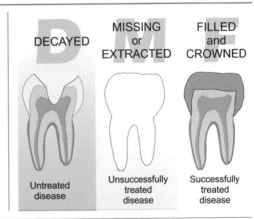

DECAYED — **MISSING** or **EXTRACTED** — **FILLED** and **CROWNED**

Untreated disease — Unsuccessfully treated disease — Successfully treated disease

There are 6 main shortcomings in using the DMF Index:

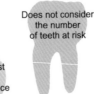

Does not distinguish between different dental health status

Not reversible

Does not consider the number of teeth at risk

Obscures the role of social factors in dental disease variation

Related to past and present caries experience

Assumes filled teeth were once decayed

EPIDEMIOLOGY OF DENTAL CARIES (2)

Trends

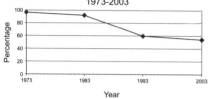

Trends in dental caries in 15-year-old children in England, 1973-2003

The percentage of 15-year-old children with dental caries has declined from 97% in 1973 to 55% in 2003. The largest drop was between 1983 and 1993. The number of caries free children is increasing.

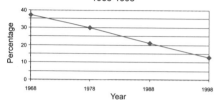

Trends in the proportion of edentulous adults in the UK, 1968-1998

The proportion of edentulous adults in the UK has declined since 1968 (Kelly et al., 2000; Gray et al., 1970). The older the individual the greater the level of edentulousness, however, this trend seems to be reducing.

Prevalence

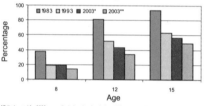

Proportion of children with obvious decay experience in permanent teeth by age in UK, 1983-2003

*Criteria used for 2003 survey (includes visual caries) **Criteria used for 1993 survey (excludes visual caries)

The proportion of children with obvious decay experience in permanent teeth has decreased in all age groups since 1983. Decay increases with age and has done so since 1983 (Pitts and Harker, 2003).

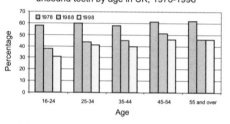

Proportion of dentate adults with some decayed or unsound teeth by age in UK, 1978-1998

Overall, the average number of decayed or unsound teeth in dentate adults decreased between 1978 and 1988, but did not change significantly between 1988 and 1998 (Walker and Cooper, 1998).

Global Goals for 2020

Hobdell and colleagues (2003) produced a document to act as an instrument for local and national health care planners to specify realistic goals and standards for oral health to be achieved by the year 2020. By being focused broadly on the global level, it is hoped that it will encourage local action in the spirit of the United Nations Development Programme's report: *'Think globally act locally'.*

GLOBAL GOALS FOR 2020: DENTAL CARIES

- To increase the proportion of caries-free 6-year-olds by X%
- To reduce the DMFT, particularly the D component, at age 12 years by X%, with special attention to high-risk groups within populations, utilising both distributions and means
- To reduce the number of teeth extracted due to dental caries at ages 18, 35-44 and 65-74 years by X%

Determinants

The major determinant of caries is sugar. However, there were other factors related to caries decline in the past decades as follows:

1982 First International Conference on the Decline in Prevalence of Dental Caries. It was suggested that the use of fluoride provides the best possible single explanation for the decline. Delegates also proposed that the overall drop is associated with several factors, some of which are unknown.

1984 Sheiham reiterated that the reduction in dental caries is likely to be multi-factorial.

1995 The FDI/WHO study suggested the following four factors:
1. Widespread exposure to fluorides
2. Provision of preventive oral health services
3. Increased dental awareness through organised oral health education programmes
4. Availability of dental resources

1995 Nadanovsky and Sheiham recognised that socio-economic factors were especially important in industrialised countries

2001 Marcenes et al. showed that changes in the diagnosis and treatment criteria have greatly contributed to a decline in caries.

Individuals At Risk

Risk factors for edentulousness include increasing age, female gender, manual occupations and living in deprived areas.

EPIDEMIOLOGY OF PERIODONTAL DISEASE (1)

Definition

Periodontal disease is not a single disease, it is however a term that covers several diseases which have proved difficult to classify. Unfortunately, in periodontal research, uniform criteria have not yet been established (Papapanou, 1996).

Clinical Diagnosis

The abbreviated version of the 1999 classification of periodontal diseases and conditions is shown below (Wiebe and Putnins, 2000):

Classification of Periodontal Diseases and Conditions

I. Gingival Diseases
    A. Dental plaque-induced gingival diseases
    B. Non-plaque-induced gingival lesions

II. Chronic Periodontitis (slight: 1-2mm Clinical Attachment Loss (CAL); moderate: 3-4mm CAL; severe: > 5mm CAL)
    A. Localised
    B. Generalised (> 30% of sites are involved)

III. Aggressive Periodontitis (slight: 1-2mm CAL; moderate: 3-4mm CAL; severe: > 5mm CAL)
    A. Localised
    B. Generalised (> 30% of sites are involved)

IV. Periodontitis as a Manifestation of Systemic Diseases
    A. Associated with haematological disorders
    B. Associated with genetic disorders
    C. Not otherwise specified

V. Necrotising Periodontal Diseases
    A. Necrotising ulcerative gingivitis
    B. Necrotising ulcerative periodontitis

VI. Abscesses of the Periodontium
    A. Gingival abscess
    B. Periodontal abscess
    C. Pericoronal abscess

VII. Periodontitis Associated With Endodontic Lesions
    A. Combined periodontic-endodontic lesions

VIII. Developmental or Acquired Deformities and Conditions
    A. Localised tooth-related factors that modify or predispose to plaque-induced gingival diseases/periodontitis
    B. Mucogingival deformities and conditions around teeth
    C. Mucogingival deformities and conditions on edentulous ridges
    D. Occlusal trauma

The bases for the definition of periodontal disease are as follows:

1. Inflammation
2. Bleeding on probing
3. Pocket formation
4. Loss of periodontal attachment
5. Loss of alveolar bone
6. Tooth mobility
7. Tooth loss

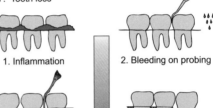

1. Inflammation

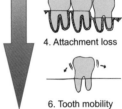

2. Bleeding on probing

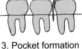

3. Pocket formation

4. Attachment loss

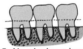

5. Alveolar bone loss

6. Tooth mobility

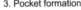

7. Tooth loss

Measures And Shortcomings

The measures of periodontal disease include:
1. **Loss of periodontal attachment**
2. **Community Periodontal Index (CPI)**
3. **Bleeding index**
4. **Pocket depths**

CPI can be used to give an indication of the periodontal status of a community. It can be used to determine changes in a population's periodontal condition, and may give an indication of success or otherwise in periodontal therapy. It can be used as a simple record keeping measure of periodontal health.

The limitations of periodontal indices are that they are prone to a high degree of subjective variability. Probing accuracy is affected by probe angulation, the amount of pressure applied, the presence of calculus and inflammation. It should also be noted that the indices do not differentiate between acute/chronic or active/inactive stages of disease (refer to Chapter 2: Epidemiology of Dental Caries for information on indices).

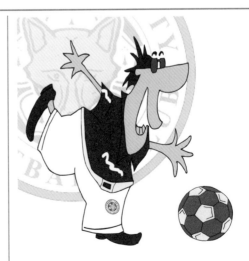

 Remember: **L**eicester **C**ity foot**B**all **P**layers... tackle periodontal disease!

EPIDEMIOLOGY OF PERIODONTAL DISEASE (2)

Trends and Prevalence

Fifty-four percent of dentate adults had pocketing of 4mm or more on at least one tooth, while 5% had some deep pocketing of 6mm or more. One third (34%) of dentate adults aged 16-24 years and nearly half (47%) of those aged 25-34 had some pocketing. These proportions increased with age up to 67% of those aged 65+ with pockets of 4mm or greater. Deep pocketing (of 6mm or more) affected a much smaller proportion of the dentate population (5%) and varied from 1% of the youngest age group up to 15% of those aged 65+ (Walker and Cooper, 1998).

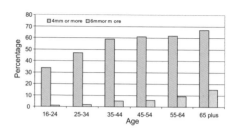

Forty-three percent of dentate adults had loss of attachment of 4mm or more around at least one tooth. This increased with age from 14% among dentate adults aged 16-24 years to 85% among those aged 65+. The proportion of dentate adults with extensive loss of attachment (of 6mm or more) also increased with age, particularly among those aged 45+. None of those aged 16-24 years had any extensive loss of attachment but nearly one-third (31%) of dentate adults aged 65+ had 6mm or more.

Proportion of dentate adults with loss of attachment of 4mm or more by age in UK

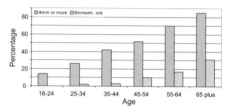

Global Goals for 2020

Hobdell and colleagues (2003) produced a document to act as an instrument for local and national health care planners to specify realistic goals and standards for oral health to be achieved by the year 2020. By being focused broadly on the global level, it is hoped that it will encourage local action in the spirit of the United Nations Development Programme's report: *'Think globally act locally'*.

GLOBAL GOALS FOR 2020: PERIODONTAL DISEASE

- To reduce the number of teeth lost due to periodontal disease by X% at ages 18, 35-44 and 65-74 years with special reference to smoking, poor oral hygiene, stress and inter-current systemic disease.
- To reduce the prevalence of necrotising forms of periodontal disease by X% by reducing exposure to risk factors such as poor nutrition, stress and immunosuppression.
- To reduce the prevalence of active periodontal infection (with or without loss of attachment) in all ages by X%.
- To increase the proportion of people in all ages with healthy periodontium (gums and supporting bone structure) by X%.

Determinants

History of the understanding of periodontal disease:

First Era
Periodontal disease was also known as **pyorrhoea**. The causes were believed to be bacterial infection, mechanical irritation, nutritional deficiencies or manifestations of systemic illness. The treatment would be extractions which would result in edentulousness.

Second Era
People believed periodontal disease was related to a patient's age, sex, socio-economic status, race or the extent of calculus and plaque deposits. It was believed that everyone was susceptible to severe periodontal disease if oral hygiene was inadequate. They felt that the **disease progressed in a linear fashion** throughout life from gingivitis to periodontitis to bone loss and eventual tooth loss. Also, that periodontal disease was the main cause of tooth loss in people aged 35 or older.

Third Era
Everything we knew about periodontal disease changed in this era. We stopped analysing data with respect to the whole mouth and concentrated on analysing data with respect to the site. This gave us a better understanding of the aetiology of periodontal disease. Now, the understanding is that most adults exhibit some gingivitis and/or mild periodontitis, but severe periodontitis is rare, even if oral hygiene is inadequate. Periodontitis **progresses by acute bursts of activity** and most gingivitis does not progress to periodontitis (Goodson *et al.*,1982; Socransky *et al.*, 1984). Caries, but not periodontal disease, is the main cause of tooth loss in adults.

Periodontal disease is complex with bacterial plaque and host susceptibility playing important roles in the occurrence of the disease.

Individuals At Risk

The people most likely to suffer from periodontal disease are older adults as the disease process is cumulative. Other at-risk groups include males, those in manual occupations, increasing stress levels and deprived communities.

EPIDEMIOLOGY OF TRAUMATIC DENTAL INJURIES (1)

Definition

Trauma is an injury that occurs suddenly and unexpectedly. Therefore it follows that the patient who has experienced the trauma is likely to be distressed and upset, as will the parents in the case of a child.

Public Health Aspects

Traumatic dental injuries are low in prevalence however, the pain and discomfort that follow are significant and there is usually some degree of functional and social limitation. Nevertheless, these injuries are treatable and more importantly preventable through public health measures, but a limiting factor is the high financial cost involved.

Public health issues related to TDIs

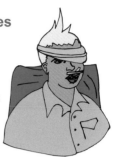

Treatable and preventable
Reduced prevalence
Agony: pain and discomfort
Useless: functional limitation
Money: financial cost
Afraid to socialise

 Remember: Public health issues related to **TRAUMA**tic dental injuries

Clinical Diagnosis

Several classifications of traumatic dental injuries (TDI) exist, though many are adapted from the WHO classification. The classification below describes injuries in terms of anatomy (Glendor *et al.*, 2006).

Hard Dental Tissue & Pulp	Periodontal Tissues	Supporting Bone	Gingiva/Oral Mucosa
• Enamel infraction • Enamel fracture • Enamel-dentin fracture • Complicated crown fracture* • Uncomplicated crown-root fracture • Complicated crown-root fracture* • Root fracture	• Concussion • Subluxation (loosening) • Extrusive luxation (peripheral dislocation, partial avulsion) • Lateral luxation • Avulsion • Intrusive luxation (central dislocation)	• Comminution of alveolar socket • Fracture of alveolar socket wall • Fracture of alveolar process • Fracture of mandible or maxilla (jaw fracture)	• Laceration of gingiva or oral mucosa • Contusion of gingiva or oral mucosa • Abrasion of gingiva or oral mucosa

* examples include complicated fractures with pulp exposure

Measures And Shortcomings

The classification above lends itself to be used in dental surgery with diagnostic aids such as pulpal sensibility tests, transillumination and radiographic examination.

Despite numerous studies on TDI it is difficult to quantify uncommon injuries as these are often omitted. In addition those injuries affecting supporting structures which leave no visible permanent marker are often not recorded. Finally, many injuries are not brought to the attention of a dentist and as a result the prevalence of TDI tends to be a gross underestimation.

Trends

The trends in TDI are not as clear-cut as those for dental caries. Studies from the UK, USA and Scandinavia suggest that there has not been a significant change in TDI. Some of the variation between the countries may be accounted for by variation in measuring TDI. It seems that the prevalence of dental caries is falling more rapidly than that of TDI. If this continues TDI may become more prevalent than dental caries (Glendor *et al.*, 2006).

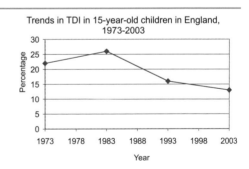

Trends in TDI in 15-year-old children in England, 1973-2003

Prevalence

The prevalence of TDIs is probably grossly underestimated in cross-sectional surveys because registration of damage depends upon clinical evidence or information from either the child or parents. It is estimated that dental trauma affects approximately 50% of school children before they reach school leaving age (Andreason, 1989). One in 4 adults and 1 in 5 children have evidence of dental injuries to permanent anterior teeth.

Age Group	Male	Female
AT 5 YEARS OF AGE (Primary dentition)	31-40%	12-33%
AT 12 YEARS OF AGE (Secondary dentition)	16-30%	4-19%
30 YEARS OLD	TDI decrease at 30 years of age	

EPIDEMIOLOGY OF TRAUMATIC DENTAL INJURIES (2)

Global Goals for 2020

Hobdell and colleagues (2003) produced a document to act as an instrument for local and national health care planners to specify realistic goals and standards for oral health to be achieved by the year 2020. By being focused broadly on the global level, it is hoped that it will encourage local action in the spirit of the United Nations Development Programme's report: *'Think globally act locally'*.

> **GLOBAL GOALS FOR 2020: TRAUMATIC DENTAL INJURIES**
> - To increase early detection by X%.
> - To increase rapid referral by X%.
> - To increase the number of health care providers who are competent to diagnose and provide emergency care by X%.
> - To increase by X% the number of affected individuals receiving multi-disciplinary specialist care where necessary.

Determinants

The determinants of TDI can be classified as:

Accidental Injuries (commonest cause of TDI)
- *Falls and collisions:* Falls from tripping, sliding, heights and from playground equipment
- *Traffic accidents:* Car, bicycle, motorcycle and pedestrian
- *Group sports:* Ice-hockey, field-hockey, basketball, rugby and football
- *Individual sports:* Snow skiing, water skiing, skateboarding, roller-skating, horse riding and swimming
- *Attack of illness:* Epilepsy and cerebral palsy

ACCIDENTAL INJURIES

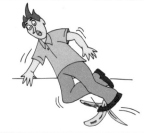

Non-Accidental Injuries
Four children die each day in the UK through non-accidental injury or neglect. 4.2 out of 1,000 children in the UK have been physically abused (Golder, 1995). In 1994 Graitcer found over 50% of all damage due to physical abuse occurs in the head and neck region. However, it should be remembered that not all oro-facial injuries are due to physical abuse. But it should be suspected if:
- There is a delay in seeking treatment
- Evidence of repetitive occurrences
- Inconsistent reporting of the cause of the injury
- History incompatible with the injury
- Vague history
- Previous history of abuse

NON-ACCIDENTAL INJURIES

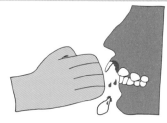

Iatrogenesis
This describes a condition that has resulted from treatment, as either an unforeseen or inevitable side-effect. An example would include injury to teeth during intubation.

IATROGENESIS

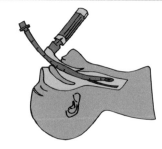

Individuals At Risk

- **Age:** Peak incidence of dental injuries at 2-4 and 8-10 years of age with a marked decrease at around 30 years of age
- **Gender:** Males at increased risk
- **Socio-economic Group:** Increased risk in higher socio-economic background (may be due to increased access to sporting activities)
- **Biological Predisposing Factors:** Increased overjet, protrusion of upper incisors and insufficient lip closure
- **Other Predisposing Factors:** Falls, traffic accidents and sports
- **Medical Illnesses:** Epilepsy and cerebral palsy

Incidence of TDI with age

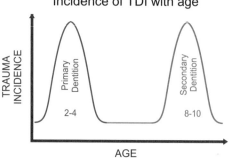

TRAUMA INCIDENCE — AGE — Primary Dentition 2-4 — Secondary Dentition 8-10

QUESTIONS

Short Answer Questions

1. What do you understand by the term 'epidemiology'? (1 mark)
2. Explain the difference between 'descriptive' and 'analytical' epidemiology and indicate the primary purpose of both types. (2 marks)
3. What is the CPIT index? Give three limitations that the CPIT index has when used to estimate periodontal treatment needs. (4 marks)
4. Name two other social background factors, in addition to age and sex, which might impact on periodontal health. (2 marks)
5. What do you understand by the term 'index'? (1 mark)
6. List and explain four criteria used to assess an epidemiological index. (3 marks)
7. What do you understand by the term 'calibration' when used in the context of a programme for an epidemiological exercise? (1 mark)
8. List two roles for a 'gold standard' examiner in a training programme. (1 mark)
9. What does the systemic review of the literature process involve? (1 mark)
10. How does a systemic review of the literature differ from a meta-analysis of the literature? (1 mark)
11. What do you understand by the term 'prevalence'? (1 mark)
12. List two biological predisposing factors to traumatic dental injuries (TDI). (1 mark)
13. Describe variations in traumatic dental injuries (TDI) by gender and social class in the UK. (2 marks)
14. List 4 environmental causes of traumatic dental injuries (TDI). (2 marks)

Long Answer Questions

Write short notes on the following topics. Up to 4 marks will be awarded for your answer.
1. Name a recognised epidemiological index to evaluate dental caries experience. Briefly describe four positive and four negative features of this index.
2. The main reasons for the observed decline in dental caries in industrialised countries.
3. The main features of clinical trials and their advantages as a research design.
4. The process of conducting an epidemiological survey.

Essay Questions

You will be awarded up to 20 marks for your answer.
1. Describe the trends in dental caries for children in the UK and the implications of these trends for dental services.
2. Describe the evidence concerning the role of dietary sugars as a cause of dental caries. What are the implications of this evidence for the prevention of dental decay in children?
3. List and describe the detailed steps you would take to conduct a survey to assess the dental health status and perceived treatment needs of Bangladeshi adults who attend general medical practices.

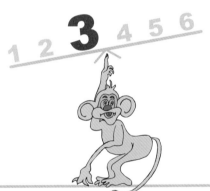

Health Promotion

CHAPTER 3

3

AIMS AND OBJECTIVES

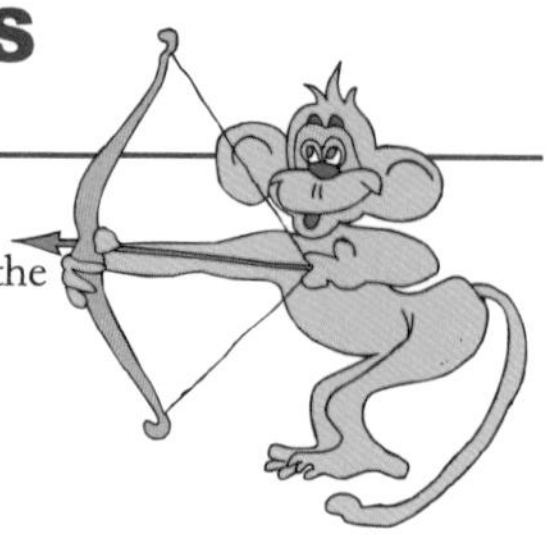

Determinants Of Health

Aim

To understand that changing definitions of health reflect a greater awareness of the range of factors which may impact upon health

Objectives
- List the factors which affect health
- Describe the key ideas of Dubos, Illich and McKeown
- Discuss research evaluating the impact of these factors
- Assess the implications of this research for improving oral health

The Concept Of Health Promotion

Aim

To understand the concept of health promotion

Objectives
- Define health promotion
- Describe the advantages of the common risk factor approach with examples
- Describe the Health Promotion Logo

Health Education

Aim

To introduce the key principles of health education

Objectives
- Define health education
- Distinguish between 'formal' and 'informal' health work
- List the current self-care messages offered to the public on the prevention of dental disease
- Explain the content of the acronym SMARTIS
- Propose some principles for improving patient education

Behaviour Change And Behaviour Change Models

Aim

To introduce the concept of behaviour change

Objectives
- List the barriers to change
- Define 'self-efficacy' and 'locus of control'
- Describe two models of behaviour change

Evaluation

Aim

To introduce valuable ways of checking activities

Objectives
- Assess the importance of evaluation
- Describe the difference between 'outcome' and 'process' evaluation
- Identify alternative methods of evaluation for different health education goals
- List three ways of conducting a process evaluation

DETERMINANTS OF HEALTH (1)

Definition

Health determinants are defined as the range of personal, social, economic and environmental factors which determine the health status of individuals or populations (Nutbeam, 1998). The factors which influence health are numerous and interactive.

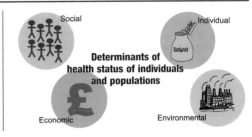

Health Fields

Lalonde (1974) described 4 key factors:

- **Personal Behaviour:** Patients should be encouraged to help themselves (e.g. regular exercise, healthy eating and brushing their teeth twice a day with fluoridated toothpaste)
- **Social and Physical Environment:** This includes factors such as pollution, overcrowding, job opportunities, locally available facilities and the quality of housing
- **Health Service:** Access to appropriate health service
- **Human Biology:** This is a non-modifiable factor

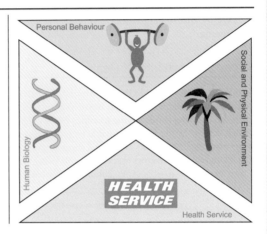

Ideas For Healthy Living

Dubos, Illich and McKeown presented their ideas for healthy living:

- **Illich (1976):** Illich proposed that better nutrition leads to an improvement in host resistance. He suggests that more self-care among lay people and minimal professional intervention will provide the best health conditions.

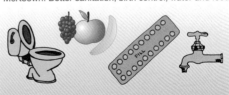

Illich: Better nutrition and less professional help

- **Dubos (1979):** Dubos believed that a healthy equilibrium is achieved by living in harmony with the external environment. Perfect health is an unattainable 'mirage'.

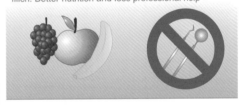

Dubos: Harmony with environment

- **McKeown (1979):** McKeown showed that mortality rate declined primarily due to better sanitation, birth control methods, water and food supply. Medicine played only a small part. He believed that successful medicine would involve not only treatment but also prevention of disease.

In 1978 the **Alma Ata Declaration** was signed. The declaration set an agenda, 'Health for all by year 2000'. At the conference the need was expressed for urgent action by all governments, all health and development workers, and the world community to protect and promote the health of all the people of the world.

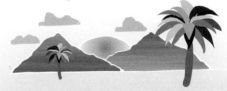

McKeown: Better sanitation, birth control, water and food

DETERMINANTS OF HEALTH (2)

Prerequisites For Health

The prerequisites for health were discussed at the First International Conference on Health Promotion in Ottawa, Canada. Improvements in health require a stable grounding in the basic prerequisites of health. These fundamental conditions and resources are listed below (WHO, 1986):

- **P**eace
- **R**esources (sustainable)
- **E**ducation
- **R**ations (food)
- **E**cosystem (stable)
- e**QU**ity and social justice
- **I**ncome
- **S**helter

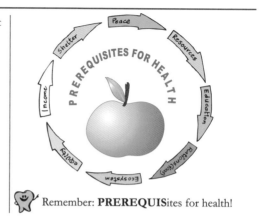

Remember: **PREREQUIS**ites for health!

Wider Determinants Of Health

Dahlgren and Whitehead (1993) portrayed the determinants of health in a visual format of concentric circles radiating outwards. The diagram below presents the determinants of health in layers of influence, starting with the individual and moving to wider society. The inner core represents the individual lifestyle factors which consist of the non-modifiable health determinants (age, gender, ethnicity and genetics). The next layer comprises social networks and social support that can affect an individual's health. The third layer consists of the more structural factors associated with living and working conditions. Finally, the outermost layer is made up of general socio-economic, cultural and environmental factors.

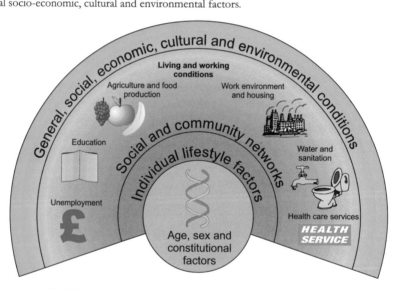

Diagram adapted from Dahlgren and Whitehead, 1993. Adapted and reproduced with permission (see Permissions).

Health Inequalities

Health inequalities are avoidable and unfair. Addressing them is a top priority for the government. Evidence shows that health inequalities have always existed. Townsend and Davidson (1982) illustrated that people of the poorest section of society receive the poorest health care. Later, Acheson (1998) showed the health inequality gap between rich and poor to be widening.

Behaviour cannot be separated from its social context. Social deprivation is linked to poor diet, less frequent oral hygiene and increased sugar consumption.

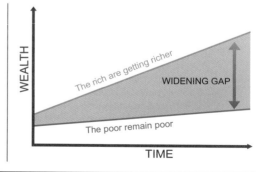

THE CONCEPT OF HEALTH PROMOTION

Definition

WHO (1984) defines *health promotion* as the process of enabling individuals and communities to increase control over the determinants of their health and thereby improve their health.

Common Risk Factor Approach

Many oral health programmes are developed and implemented in isolation from other health programmes. At best this leads to a duplication of efforts and at worst conflicting messages (Sheiham and Watt, 2000).

The common risk factor approach (CRFA) maximises resources by targeting risk factors common to many chronic conditions, as many risk factors are related to more than one condition.

A good example is 'smoking' as it is linked to many diseases (e.g. diabetes, cancers, cardiovascular, respiratory and periodontal diseases). The CRFA promotes general health by controlling a small number of risk factors. It also has an impact on a number of different diseases at a lower cost. The diagram opposite illustrates examples.

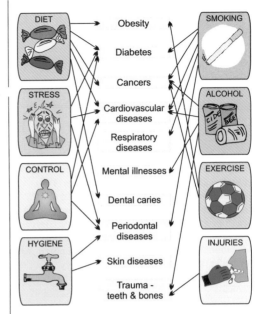

Diagram adapted from Sheiham and Watt, 2000. Adapted and reproduced with permission (see Permissions).

Health Promotion Logo

The health promotion logo was created at the First International Conference on Health Promotion in Ottawa, Canada. The logo is made up of an outer circle within which there are 3 wings that originate from an inner spot. One of the wings breaks through the outer circle. The logo integrates **5 key action areas in health promotion** and **3 basic health promotion strategies** (see diagram below for details). The health promotion strategies are advocacy for health; enabling people to achieve their full health potential; and mediating between the different interests in society in pursuit of health (WHO, 1986).

Strengthen community action: Health promotion works through concrete and effective community work in setting priorities, making decisions, planning strategies and implementing them to achieve better health. The centre of this process is empowerment of communities, their ownership and control of their own endeavours and destinies.

Reorient health services: The responsibility for health promotion in health services is divided among individuals, community groups, health professionals, health service institutes and governments. They must all work together towards a health care system which contributes to the pursuit of health. The health sector must move increasingly in the health promotion direction, over its responsibility for providing clinical and curative services.

Building healthy public policies: This is represented by the outside circle, which symbolises the need for policies to 'hold things together'. Health promotion places health on the agenda of policy makers of all sectors and at all levels. It alerts them to the health consequences of their decisions and to accept their responsibilities for health. It should unite various approaches such as legislation, taxation and organisational changes to bring about safer and healthier goods and services, healthier public service, and cleaner, more enjoyable environments.

Develop personal skills: Health promotion supports personal and social development by providing information and health education and enhancing life skills. It increases the options available for people to exercise. This allows them more control over their own health and their environment. Overall, it allows healthier choices conducive to health.

Create supportive environments: There are inextricable links between people and their environment, which constitute the basis for a socio-ecological approach to health. Reciprocal maintenance should be the guiding message to all to take care of each other, our communities and our natural environment. In the rapidly changing environment society must organise work to help create a healthy society.

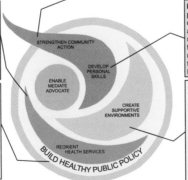

Diagram adapted from WHO, 1986. Adapted and reproduced with permission (see Permissions).

Types Of Health Service

- **Personal Health Services** are those provided directly by the provider to the patient (e.g. reassurance and treatment of emergencies).
- **Non-Personal Health Services** are those services made available to the public at large through other agencies (e.g. water fluoridation) (McKeown, 1979).

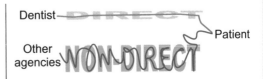

HEALTH EDUCATION (1)

Definition

Health education is centred around creating opportunities for learning, specifically aimed at producing a health-related goal (WHO, 1984). Health education gives knowledge, develops skills, ensures understanding of health issues and promotes self-esteem. These are essential ingredients for health promotion, as they attempt to improve an individual's ability to choose a healthier lifestyle.

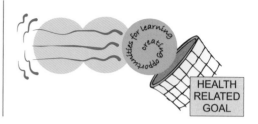

Key Principles

Knowledge should be given to ensure understanding and promote self-esteem. The information should be given in a value-free and unbiased manner. The educator's ideas should not be imposed on the patients (i.e. must be voluntarist). The outcomes of health education should be to increase awareness and knowledge. This can be done through personal education (i.e. dentist/patient, teacher/pupil) or mass media (i.e. public relations, advertising, news, World Wide Web). However, it is important to stress that knowledge does not necessarily lead to behaviour change and that inadequate resources may be a limiting factor.

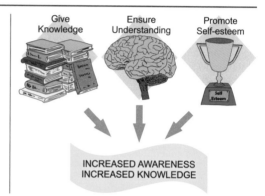

Health Work

Health related work may be:

- **Formal:** That provided by the health care professionals, who have undergone specialist training and are paid for their work (e.g. the primary dental care team).

- **Informal:** Those people contributing to the maintenance of health and providing care during illness (e.g. self-care, family care, community self-help groups). This makes up approximately 75-85% of all health care efforts.

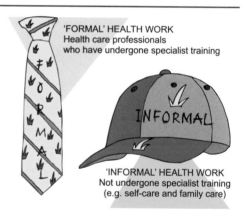

Classification

Health education may lead to the prevention of dental disease. Health education can be classified into population-based (primary) and patient-based (secondary and tertiary):
- **Primary:** Preventing ill-health arising (population-based)
- **Secondary:** Preventing ill-health becoming chronic/irreversible (patient-based)
- **Tertiary:** Helping people make the most of the remaining potential for healthy living, avoiding unnecessary hardship and complications (patient-based)

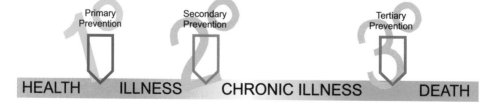

HEALTH EDUCATION (2)

Advice To The Public

A policy document produced by the Health Development Agency refined and standardised the advice given to the public. It ensured that the recommendations were scientifically sound. Advice to the public should be based on the following clear and simple statements (Levine, 2001):

1. Diet: Reduce the consumption and especially the frequency of intake of foods and drinks with added sugars. The frequency of sugars entering the mouth is an important factor in determining the rate of tooth decay, therefore snacking between meals should be avoided. Acidic drinks including squashes and carbonated drinks are particularly detrimental.

2. Tooth brushing: Clean teeth thoroughly twice daily with a fluoride toothpaste. Tooth brushing is essential to remove plaque and prevent periodontal disease. It is important to emphasise that thorough brushing of all tooth surfaces and gum margins twice a day is more important than more frequent cursory brushing.

3. Fluoridation: Water fluoridation is a safe and effective public health measure. This is considered to be the most effective, safe and efficient public health measure for reducing dental caries. The optimum level is one part of fluoride per million water (1 ppm).

4. Dental Attendance: Have an oral examination by a dentist every year. Those at risk from oral disease such as children may need more frequent visits.

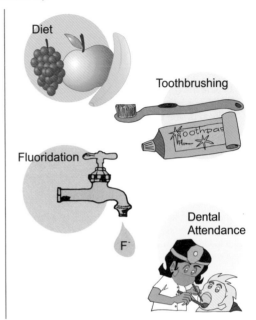

Dental health education must be approached with the same dedication which is applied to the treatment of dental disease.

'SMARTIS' Objectives

Successful health education planning requires the use of aims (set out goals) and objectives (specific targets).

Aim: Broad general statement of what you want to achieve (e.g. to make health information available).

Objective: Specific end result to be achieved within a specific time period (e.g. to distribute six leaflets to 25 dental surgeries within three months).

 Remember: In order for an objective to be useful, remember **SMART** (Jacob and Plamping, 1989), or **SMARTIS**

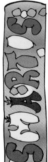

Specific: Concrete, detailed, focused and well defined objective

Measurable: Measurement source identified and allows follow-up of progress

Appropriate: Suitable objective

Realistic: Objective is achievable with the resources available

Time-Related: Setting deadlines for the achievement of the objective

Important: Objective is significant to the patient

Support: Encourage the patient

General and Specific Factors For Successful Health Education

General Factors
Oral health education can be delivered through various sources such as posters, leaflets, audio-visual aids, oral presentations and the media. For oral health education to be successful it should be:

- **G** Part of a strate**G**y
- **E** **E**ncouragement and supportive participation
- **N** Seek to i**N**tegrate
- **E** Should seek an **E**arly involvement
- **R** **R**elevant and appropriate goals
- **A** **A**nxiety: to reduce
- **L** **L**ook for and adopt diverse approaches

Specific Factors
To facilitate behaviour change and compliance the following simple methods can be employed in everyday practice:

- **S** **S**tress and repeat key points
- **P** **P**recise and specific
- **E** **E**yes: visual aids
- **C** **C**oncise and realistic amount of information given
- **I** **I**mportant things first
- **F** **F**ree of jargon
- **I** 'l**i**ttle information: not too much information given
- **C** **C**ategories: structure information into categories

 Remember: The **GENERAL** and **SPECIFIC** factors for successful health education

BEHAVIOUR CHANGE

Definitions

Health behaviour is defined as any activity undertaken by an individual, regardless of actual or perceived health status, for the purpose of promoting, protecting or maintaining health, whether or not such behaviour is objectively effective towards that end (Nutbeam, 1998). Before behaviour can be changed, patients must (Chestnutt, 1998):

- Want to change
- Believe they can change
- Believe the change will have the desired effect
- Possess or be provided with the knowledge and skills to permit change

In order for the behaviour change to have a lasting effect, compliance is of the utmost importance. *Compliance* is the degree of constancy and accuracy with which a patient follows a prescribed regimen (e.g. regular flossing or avoidance of sugary snacks). Although we often talk of compliance with our regimens, what we should be talking of is *concordance*. Concordance recognises the central role patient participation has in all good care plans (Longmore *et al.*, 2004).

Self-efficacy is a belief in one's own ability to bring about a behaviour change effectively (Bandura, 1977). If change is not started because of fear of failing you have low self-efficacy (i.e. a low self-estimation of the ability to change). This can be developed by verbal persuasion, learning from experience and successful practice.

Locus of Control describes perceived control over outcomes (Wallston *et al.*, 1978). There are three classifications:

- **Internal:** a belief that personal action can lead to health outcomes
- **External/Chance:** health outcomes are largely controlled by fate
- **Powerful Others:** behaviour is in the hands of

HEALTH BEHAVIOUR

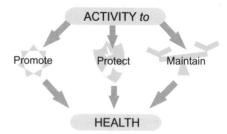

SELF-EFFICACY

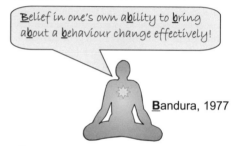

Belief in one's own ability to bring about a behaviour change effectively!

Bandura, 1977

Remember: The **B**'s in **B**anduras definition of self-efficacy

LOCUS OF CONTROL

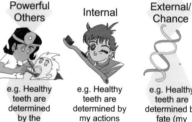

Powerful Others	Internal	External/Chance
e.g. Healthy teeth are determined by the Dentist	e.g. Healthy teeth are determined by my actions (toothbrushing)	e.g. Healthy teeth are determined by fate (my genes)

Barriers To Change

There are many barriers that hinder individuals from changing their health-related practices. These arise from internal factors within the individual or are related to external socio-environmental factors. They are:

- **Belief** that people cannot change
- **Anxiety** about getting the change wrong
- **Difficult nature of change**, intrusive or time consuming
- **Bloody uncertain** consequences (and slow)
- **Awareness** and knowledge about how to change
- **Resources**: Lack of
- **Rival**/Conflicting motives
- **Inherited**: Belief that it is all genetic so there is no point in changing
- **Effort** needed continuously, rather than a one-off
- **UnRealistic** targets
- **Satisfy** someone else

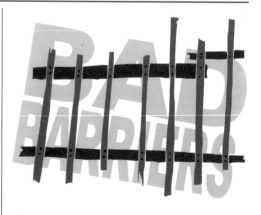

Remember: the **BAD BARRIERS** to change

BEHAVIOUR CHANGE MODELS

Model 1: Change Model

The stages of the Transtheoretical Change Model are presented below (Prochaska and DiClemente, 1983). The stages in the change model are linked together in a cycle of change and they are not simply related in a straight line fashion. There is a need to identify where the patient is on the cycle of change before interventions can take place. Other factors that influence the cycle include self-efficacy and locus of control.

Stage	Patient's Role	Health Educator's Role
Pre-contemplation	There is no consideration for behaviour change	Need to increase knowledge and awareness
Contemplation	Thinking over the pros and cons of behaviour change	Motivation and negotiation
Preparation	Making definite plans to change	Assistance
Action	The actual behaviour change is started	Setting goals - SMARTIS
Maintenance	The active sustaining of behaviour change	Feedback, monitoring and rewards

A Case Study

Watt (1997) carried out a study which examined the stages of change for sugar and fat reduction in an adolescent sample.

Sample: 479 (13-14 year old) children attending four London secondary schools were examined.

Results: Low proportions were in contemplation or preparation stages for either fat or sugar consumption change. Higher proportions were in pre-contemplation, action or maintenance stages. Males were more likely to be at pre-contemplation stage, whereas females were more likely to be in contemplation or action stages.

Discussion: It was found that social and structural factors were important in influencing eating patterns (e.g. availability, cost, food labelling). This study has identified that different support strategies are needed for males and females as they are at different stages of the change model. This will enable appropriate targeting of their needs.

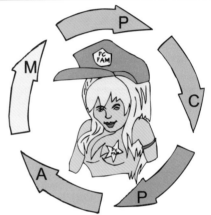

 Remember: **PC PAM**ela - A super-model who *changed* when she had plastic surgery!

Model 2: The Precede-Proceed Model

This model provides a tool to deliver a health education programme and also evaluates its ability to meet its goals (Green and Kreuter, 1991). The model consists of 9 phases:

- **Phase 1:** Identify health goals of the target population
- **Phase 2:** Identify the oral health-related problems of the population
- **Phase 3:** Identify the specific influences on the chosen oral health problem (including environmental and behavioural factors)
- **Phase 4:** Investigate the factors which influence behaviour change (e.g. predisposing attitudes or beliefs)
- **Phase 5:** Issues in implementing a programme (e.g. facilities, expertise, cost)
- **Phase 6:** Implementation and re-evaluation
- **Phase 7:** Process evaluation to see if educational and organisational factors were successful
- **Phase 8:** Impact evaluation to see if behavioural and environmental factors were successfully changed
- **Phase 9:** The final stage evaluates the overall outcomes by change towards health goals and improved health

1. Health goals

2. Oral health-related problems

3. Influences on the problem

4. Factors which influence behaviour change

5. Programme implementation

6. Implement

7. Process evaluation

8. Impact evaluation

9. Outcome evaluation

EVALUATION

Definition

Evaluation is the determination of the effectiveness, efficiency and acceptability of a planned intervention in achieving stated objectives. More specifically, *health promotion evaluation* is an assessment of the extent to which health promotion actions achieve a 'valued' outcome (Nutbeam, 1998). It is important to evaluate oral health promotion as it can be used to:

- Assess whether an activity has been achieved (dependent on aims and objectives)
- Measure the impact of an activity
- Monitor progress
- Identify strengths and weaknesses
- Plan the way ahead (e.g. staff development)

Evaluation can be divided into that related to the outcomes (summative) and that related to the process (formative).

PLANNED INTERVENTION

Effectiveness   Efficiency   Acceptability

OBJECTIVE ACHIEVED?

Outcome Evaluation

What an activity has achieved.

Outcome Evaluation is the outputs and outcomes of health promotion, the effectiveness of an activity in meeting its pre-defined objectives (e.g. the amount by which the plaque index has improved). There are three groups of indicators that can be used to assess outcome evaluation:

1. *Outcome Indicators:* The ultimate indicator (e.g. positive change in health status, reported tooth-brushing behaviour, observation of practices or changes in attitudes and knowledge)
2. *Intermediate Indicators:* Where direct measures are not possible (e.g. number of toothbrushes, amount of floss bought)
3. *Indirect Indicators:* Where direct and intermediate indicators are not possible (e.g. the number of leaflets produced, number of staff trained, sessions of oral hygiene instruction)

Difference Between Process and Outcome Evaluation

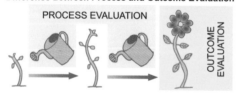

Process Evaluation

Explaining *how* outcomes have been achieved.

Process Evaluation is the feedback on what took place when a particular activity or programme was implemented and how outcomes were brought about (e.g. the roles adopted, patterns of communication by dentists). Below are several ways of conducting a process evaluation along with examples of each.

1. *Self-evaluation:* 'What did I do well?' 'How could I improve next time?'
2. *Peer-evaluation:* Feedback from trusted colleagues
3. *Client-evaluation:* Asking patients to summarise what I have taught them
4. *Record Keeping:* A legal document that allows comparisons to be made from time to time (e.g. BPE score)

Process Evaluation

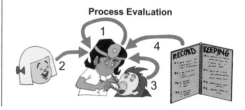

Measures Of Evaluation

The choice of evaluation measures depends on the original aims and objectives. They can be divided as follows:

1. **Health Awareness:** Measuring interest (leaflets taken, number of enquiries), change in demand for services, analysis of media coverage, questionnaires
2. **Knowledge/Attitudes:** Note changes in self-reports of clients, interviews and discussions, demonstrations of knowledge, written tests/questionnaire
3. **Behaviour Change:** Observation, recording behaviour, client demonstration
4. **Policy Change:** Policy statements and their implementation, legislation, availability of product, changes in procedures (more time for patient education)

1. Health Awareness

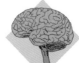

2. Knowledge/ Attitudes

3. Behaviour Change

4. Policy Change

QUESTIONS

Short Answer Questions

1. 'Health education goals negotiated with patients should be appropriate and measurable.' Explain what you understand by this statement. (1 mark)
2. List four additional criteria used when setting health education goals. (1 mark)
3. Read the following patient case history. Suggest two goals you would like to negotiate with this patient, indicating clearly how you would have used the criteria you have outlined above. *'The patient is a young woman aged 24 years. She is unemployed and living at home with her parents. She presents at the clinic with toothache, and tells you that she has several fillings and crowns. Her complaint is that the fillings dropped out and she cannot eat anything cold because her teeth are sensitive. She brushes her teeth irregularly (approximately once a week) because she finds it makes her gag. One memory she has of dental health instruction is being told to brush her teeth after eating sweets.'* (3 marks)
4. List four stages of change in the Transtheoretical Model of behaviour change. (2 marks)
5. Outline three implications of the Transtheoretical Model of behaviour change for oral health promotion. (3 marks)
6. What do you understand by the term 'health education'? (1 mark)
7. What do you understand by the term 'primary health care'? (1 mark)
8. Name two members of the UK primary health care team (other than the dental team). (1 mark)
9. Name one important theoretical advantage in the use of members of the primary health care team to promote oral health. (1 mark)
10. Give specific examples of two oral health promotion campaigns in which members of the UK primary health care team (other than the dental team) have promoted aspects of oral health. (2 marks)
11. List four factors which can be adopted to improve patient education. (2 marks)
12. What do you understand by the terms 'outcome' and 'process' evaluation? (2 marks)
13. Name one outcome and one process evaluation measure you would use for a session of patient education. (1 mark)
14. What is the definition of 'health' proposed by the World Health Organization (WHO)? (1 mark)
15. List one positive and one negative attribute of this definition. (2 marks)
16. What do you understand by the term 'self-efficacy'? (1 mark)
17. Name two theoretical models which can be used to improve the effectiveness of oral health education. (2 marks)
18. List four barriers that prevent individuals from changing their oral health behaviour. (2 marks)

Long Answer Questions

Write short notes on the following topics. Up to 4 marks will be awarded for your answer.
1. The advantages and disadvantages of oral health education leaflets.
2. The relationship between knowledge, attitudes and behaviour and its implications for oral health promotion.
3. The meaning of community participation and multi-sectorality and their contribution to health promotion activity.
4. The main features and criticisms of the Transtheoretical Model of behaviour change.
5. The criteria to be used when goal setting with patients.
6. The current consensus messages for the prevention of dental disease.
7. The Precede-Proceed Model of behaviour change.
8. The common risk factor approach (CRFA) and its application to oral conditions.
9. Formal and informal health work.
10. Process and outcome evaluations and their measurement.

Essay Questions

You will be awarded up to 20 marks for your answer.
1. What do you understand by the terms 'health education' and 'health promotion'? Describe the features of a health promotion strategy to prevent dental caries.
2. List and describe with examples the range of activities you would find within a health promotion strategy. Use this range of activities to develop the content of a health promotion programme to prevent traumatic dental injuries in children.
3. Outline the four key messages for the prevention of dental diseases and the scientific background of these messages. Use this information to propose a preventative strategy for dental caries for a child population attending a general dental practice.

MY NOTES AND SPIDERGRAM

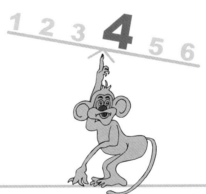

Oral Health Care

CHAPTER 4

AIMS AND OBJECTIVES

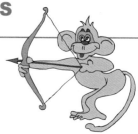

Introduction

Aim

To provide an overview of a health care system

Objectives
- Define health care system
- Analyse the features of a health care system
- Assess the factors that influence the organisation of health care

Structure Of The NHS And Dentistry

Aim

To introduce the structure and organisation of the NHS in the UK

Objectives
- Discuss the organisation of health care in the UK
- Describe the development, structure and financing of the NHS in the UK
- Describe the delivery of oral health care in the UK

Oral Health Care In The UK

Aim

To introduce the arrangements for providing dental services in the UK

Objectives
- Discuss human resources in dental care
- Discuss the training requirements for independent practice
- Describe the different methods of payment and employment of dentists/PCDs

Health Care Quality

Aim

To explore issues related to health care quality

Objectives
- Define health care and health care quality
- Describe and apply Maxwell's criteria for assessing quality in health care
- Discuss the reasons for the increasing interest in health care quality
- List the techniques and tools for achieving and managing quality

Clinical Governance

Aim

To explore clinical governance in NHS dentistry

Objectives
- Describe the features of clinical governance
- Discuss the implications of clinical governance for the GDP

Options For Change

Aim

To discuss government strategy for NHS dentistry, 'Options for Change'

Objective
- Discuss how 'Options for Change' addresses quality of oral health care

Barriers To Access

Aim

To explore the common problems with health care delivery

Objectives
- Explain the five dimensions of access
- Describe factors influencing a patient's ability to access health care facilities
- Describe the Dudley experiment
- List and evaluate methods of improving access to services

The Roadside Dentist

Aim

To appreciate a different health care system

INTRODUCTION (1)

Definitions

A *system* is a set of elements, actively interrelated, which operates within a bounded unit.

A *health system* is the totality of formal efforts, commitments, personnel, institutions, economic resources and research efforts that a nation, state or society devotes to illness, premature mortality, incapacitation, prevention, rehabilitation and other health-related problems.

A *health system* comprises all the organisations and resources that are devoted to producing health action and includes all the activities whose primary purpose is to promote, restore and maintain health (WHO).

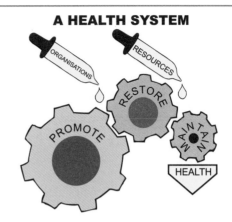

A HEALTH SYSTEM

Organisation Of Health Care

An assessment of an oral health system requires a description of who provides what services, for whom and with what resources, by what payment mechanisms and with what effect (Gift *et al.*, 1997).

The features of a health care system comprise the following factors: financial resources, operational activities (functions), service/system users (target population) and human resources.

REMEMBER

Financial resources
- How is health care funded? General taxation, National Insurance, private insurance, out-of-pocket payment or direct payment
- Where does the money come from?
- How is the money allocated?
- What are the priorities?
- Is there accountability for spending?

Operational activities
- Types of activities performed: treatment-orientated, prevention-orientated, screening and epidemiology, emergency services, professional education, health education
- Way in which health care is delivered
- Any quality control measures
- Effectiveness of the health service provided
- Efficiency of health service provided: hospitals, health centres, general practices, roadside dentists in India, barefoot dentists in China, distribution of facilities

System/ service users (target population)
- Is it equally available for all?
- Accessibility of the services
- Do the services meet consumer wants and needs?
- Waiting times
- Satisfaction with services

Human resources
- Volume: size of the workforce relative to population, recruitment
- Skills mix: types of health workers available (dentists, hygienists, therapists, nurses, technicians)
- Distribution of workforce geographically
- Remuneration methods
- Accountability for professional/ clinical performance
- Culture: values and beliefs of the workforce

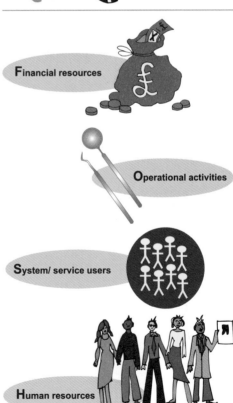

Financial resources

Operational activities

System/ service users

Human resources

 Remember: **FOSH**, not fish for organisation of health care.

INTRODUCTION (2)

Factors That Influence The Organisation Of Health Care

The organisation of health care is influenced by political, economic, social and technological factors.

Political

This is the degree and forms of state intervention, which reflect political ideas, government priorities and public opinion. The impacts on the organisation of health care are:

- Sources of finance
- Amount of financial resources
- Methods of remuneration
- Professional autonomy
- Types of services
- Types of patients
- Freedom of choice (in choosing providers)
- Changes in the internal structure and operation of the public sector competition, markets, decentralisation

Economic

- Industrialisation: health conditions become more complex with rapid growth of the private sector (e.g. in Thailand)
- Economic integration with other countries (e.g. Mexico and America leading to penetration of US health corporations)

Social

- Socio-demographic changes (e.g. rapidly ageing population, changing patterns of health needs, increasing pressure, financing)
- Socio-epidemiological changes: infectious diseases, chronic illnesses and injuries
- Educational: health knowledge, demand on services

Technological

- Identification of health problems
- Treatment of health problems
- Scientific precision in clinical practice
- Public fascination
- Symbol of success

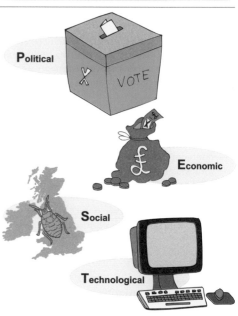

Remember: **PEST** factors influence the organisation of health care.

Summary Of FOSH And PEST

The way health care is organised in a particular society or country affects the health and quality of life of that society and has an impact on the professional life of health care workers.

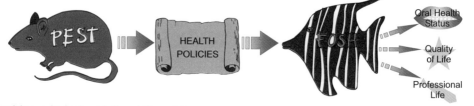

Problems In Industrialised Countries

There are a number of common problems facing oral health care systems in industrialised countries:

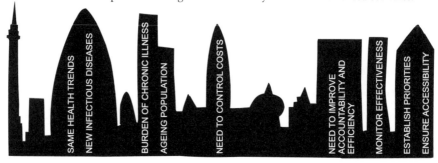

STRUCTURE OF THE NHS AND DENTISTRY (1)

Pre-NHS Health Care System

Pre-NHS health care was fragmented, with little coordination and limited access. The system depended on the ability to pay and hence there was a mismatch between geographical need and availability. Before the NHS there was a disorganised and complex mixture of private and public services:

 PUBLIC **PRIVATE**

Municipal Hospitals	Private Practitioners	Voluntary Hospitals	Voluntary and Commercial Organisations
• Poor law • Amendment Act 1834 • Workhouses to provide relief to the poor - diverse network of hospitals	• Fees charged for services • Club practice • Excluded the unemployed and their dependants	• Funded by philanthropy or public subscription • Funding decreased from 1939 • Insurance plan • Selective admissions	• Insurance companies and friendly societies involved in the financing of health care • Voluntary organisations involved in provision of community health services

The NHS

In 1948 the NHS was founded and funded by central taxation. From the beginning it was challenged by resource constraints. Hospital, consultant and specialist services consumed 70% of resources. Sixteen percent of the population sought dental treatment within the first few months. In 1951 to compensate for the unforeseen expenditure, direct charges were introduced. Although dental treatment was free, patients had to pay for half the cost of dentures. The first significant organisational change in the GDS since 1948 took place in 1990 for general dental practitioners. Patients' dental health has improved with the greater availability of services. The emphasis has shifted steadily towards conservation and prevention.

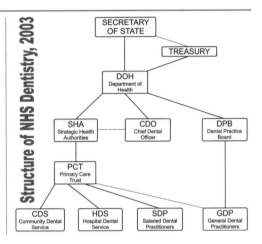

Structure of NHS Dentistry, 2003

Critical Perspectives Of Health Care Today

There are five critical perspectives of health care: the economic critique, technological pessimists, Marxist perspective, the feminist critique and iatrogenesis (Illich's thesis):

- **Illich's** thesis proposes medical interventions to be direct threats to health. These would include diagnostic errors, accidents and side-effects during treatment.

- The **Technological** pessimists feel that advances in medical technology make health care increasingly inhumane and depersonalise patient care. This increases the power of the doctor over the patient.

- The **Economic** critiques feel that health care today is inefficient and ineffective. There is variation in diagnosis and treatment, together with a tendency to over-diagnose.

- The **Marxist** suggests that health inequalities exist, with the poorest areas least likely to receive high-quality care. He feels that higher social classes get more resources relative to their level of need.

- The **Feminist** critiques feel that the delivery of health services is dominated by men and there is a failure to understand women's health care needs.

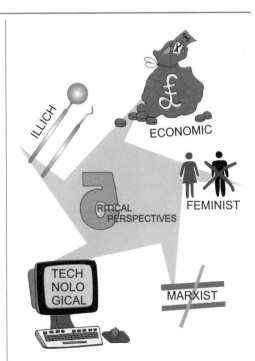

 Remember: **ITEM** Five

STRUCTURE OF THE NHS AND DENTISTRY (2)

Main Branches In Dentistry

Primary Care Trusts (PCTs) are NHS organisations whose main responsibilities are to improve the health of the community, develop primary and community health services and commission hospital care for their local population. Dental care may be accessed from the HDS, CDS, GDS, PDS and private dentistry.

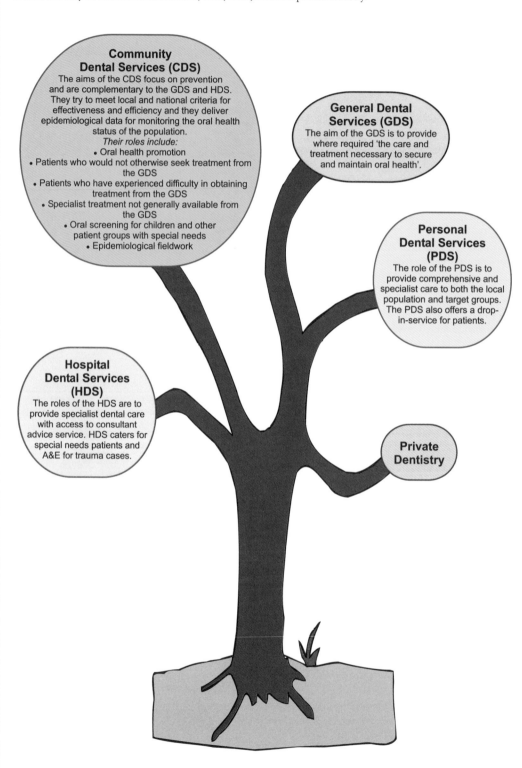

Community Dental Services (CDS)

The aims of the CDS focus on prevention and are complementary to the GDS and HDS. They try to meet local and national criteria for effectiveness and efficiency and they deliver epidemiological data for monitoring the oral health status of the population.

Their roles include:
- Oral health promotion
- Patients who would not otherwise seek treatment from the GDS
- Patients who have experienced difficulty in obtaining treatment from the GDS
- Specialist treatment not generally available from the GDS
- Oral screening for children and other patient groups with special needs
- Epidemiological fieldwork

General Dental Services (GDS)

The aim of the GDS is to provide where required 'the care and treatment necessary to secure and maintain oral health'.

Personal Dental Services (PDS)

The role of the PDS is to provide comprehensive and specialist care to both the local population and target groups. The PDS also offers a drop-in-service for patients.

Hospital Dental Services (HDS)

The roles of the HDS are to provide specialist dental care with access to consultant advice service. HDS caters for special needs patients and A&E for trauma cases.

Private Dentistry

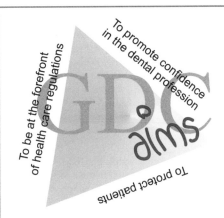

ORAL HEALTH CARE IN THE UK (1)

Continuing Professional Development

Quality of dental care provided in the UK is monitored strictly by the Dental Practice Board (DPB) and General Dental Council (GDC).

General Dental Council: Registration and re-certification are prerequisites for practice in the UK. The role of the GDC is to protect patients and to maintain the dentists' register and the roles of the professionals complementary to dentistry (PCDs). The functions of the GDC are:

- To discipline dentists and PCDs who fall short of high standards
- Suspend/limit practitioners who fall below required standards
- Publish guidance for dentists on maintaining standards and curriculum requirements
- Visit and report on UK dental and auxillary schools
- Assess postgraduate activity

Life Long Learning (LLL): A compulsory re-certification programme to promote continuing professional development (CPD). It consists of 250 hours of CPD over 5 years, of which 75 hours must be verifiable (see Clinical Governance section for more details). This requirement is mandatory for all dentists and it is their responsibility to maintain their own CPD record.

The General Dental Council monitor the scheme through random sampling and failure to comply with the regulations may lead to erasure from the dentists' register.

The reasons for its implementation are numerous. The profession is expected to be more accountable as the public is more demanding. The government strongly supports CPD with the aims of achieving excellence in clinical care and promoting a positive image of the profession.

The benefits of LLL are gained by both the patient and the dentist. For the dentist it:

- Allows more satisfaction
- Formalises existing good practice
- Creates opportunity for professional development
- Prevents boredom
- Adheres to government policy

With regard to the patient's view there is:

- Greater public protection
- Enhanced public confidence in dentistry

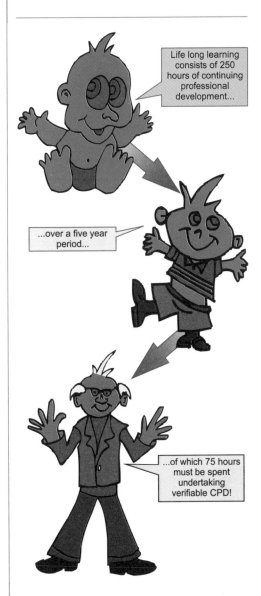

ORAL HEALTH CARE IN THE UK (2)
Vocational Training (VT) And General Professional Training (GPT)

Vocational Training (VT): This is one year of experience in practice in a supported and structured setting to ease the transition of the new graduate into general practice. The aims are to enhance clinical and administrative competence and to promote high ethical standards and care. Completion of a VT year is required for a dental graduate to enter into unsupervised NHS practice. The VT year allows new graduates to gain experience without financial pressure.

General Professional Training (GPT): This is a two-year period of structured training to further develop knowledge, skills and attitudes common to all branches of the dental profession. This will provide a basis for informed career choice and improved patient care. The GDP component must be at least one year, followed by experience of secondary care.

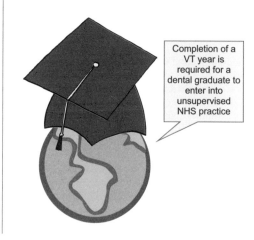

Completion of a VT year is required for a dental graduate to enter into unsupervised NHS practice

Methods Of Payment For Dental Care

The NHS is a highly complex organisation. There are four main ways dentists are remunerated for their service: fee per item, sessional, salaried and capitation.

	Advantages	Disadvantages
Fee per item	Good in areas of high need Reward for output Easy to measure No ceiling to dentist's earnings	Potential for over treatment Difficult to budget Little incentive for prevention
Sessional	Regular income Minimal administration Option for special needs/specialised care Incentive for prevention	Potential for under treatment May not treat difficult cases
Salaried	Regular income, sick pay etc. Simple administration Treatment not influenced by profit Option for special needs Incentive for prevention	Potential for under treatment Lack financial incentives to work (output) Needs extensive management
Capitation	Minimal administration Reward linked to registrations Treatment not linked to profit Incentive for prevention	Potential for under treatment May not treat difficult cases Difficult to measure output 'Unfair' in areas of high treatment need

The Dental Team

There are a number of ways in which dental care can be organised. The dental team consists of many players including dentists, dental nurses, dental hygienists, dental therapists, dental technicians, practice managers and receptionists.

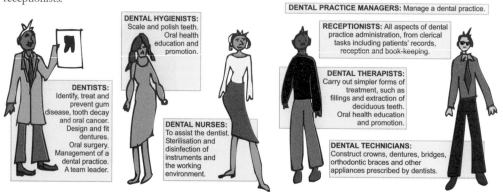

DENTAL HYGIENISTS: Scale and polish teeth. Oral health education and promotion.

DENTAL PRACTICE MANAGERS: Manage a dental practice.

RECEPTIONISTS: All aspects of dental practice administration, from clerical tasks including patients' records, reception and book-keeping.

DENTISTS: Identify, treat and prevent gum disease, tooth decay and oral cancer. Design and fit dentures. Oral surgery. Management of a dental practice. A team leader.

DENTAL THERAPISTS: Carry out simpler forms of treatment, such as fillings and extraction of deciduous teeth. Oral health education and promotion.

DENTAL NURSES: To assist the dentist. Sterilisation and disinfection of instruments and the working environment.

DENTAL TECHNICIANS: Construct crowns, dentures, bridges, orthodontic braces and other appliances prescribed by dentists.

HEALTH CARE QUALITY (1)

Definitions

Health care is defined as the health care systems and actions taken within them designed to improve health and well-being.

Health care quality can be defined in both generic and disaggregated terms. Generic definitions are often general and non-specific. For example:

- The Joint Commission on the Accreditation of Health Care Organisations defines it as the degree to which patient care services increase the probability of desired outcomes and reduce the possibility of undesired outcomes, given the current state of knowledge.
- The American Institute of Medicine defines it as the degree to which health services for individuals and populations increase the likelihood of desired health outcomes and are consistent with current professional knowledge.

Both definitions focus on excellence, zero defects and expectations or goals which have yet to be met.

Two disaggregated definitions of health care quality are described in the table below, where quality is defined according to individual components:

Maxwell (1984)*	Donabedian (1990)
Accessibility	
Relevance to need	
Social acceptability	Social acceptability
Effectiveness	Effectiveness
Equity	Equity
Efficiency	Efficiency
	Legitimacy
	Efficacy
	Optimality

* Described in detail overleaf

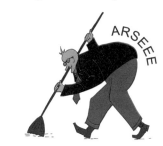

Remember: For good quality, do not be **ARSE-EE**, remember Maxwell's criteria!

Concepts Of Health Care

Health care may be conceptualised in terms of its structure, processes and outcomes (Donabedian, 1974):

Structure
This is the channel through which care is delivered and received. It is sub-divided into:
- *Organisational factors:* e.g. relationship between primary and secondary care
- *Physical:* e.g. resources (buildings, equipment), management (opening hours, booking system)
- *Staff characteristics:* e.g. skill-mix, team-working

Process
This comprises the actual care delivered and received, interactions between users and the health care structure.
- *Clinical care:* e.g. application of clinical knowledge
- *Interpersonal care:* e.g. communication skills, interpersonal skills, empathy, responsiveness, sensitivity and shared decisions about management

Outcome
This is the consequence of interactions between individuals and a health care system.
- *Health status:* e.g. functional status, symptom relief
- *User evaluation:* e.g. satisfaction, enablement (empowerment), health related quality of life

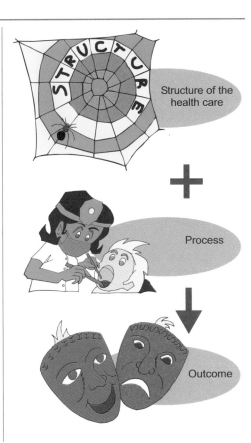

Structure of the health care

Process

Outcome

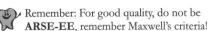

HEALTH CARE QUALITY (2)

Concepts Of Health Care Quality

Different groups of people define health care quality differently. Patients perceive quality by the amount of information given and dentists' communicating style (chair-side manner). On the other hand, the government recognises quality by measures such as efficiency (=actual output/input), cost effectiveness (=actual outcome/desired outcome) and clinical effectiveness. The GDC's bench mark for quality is competence.

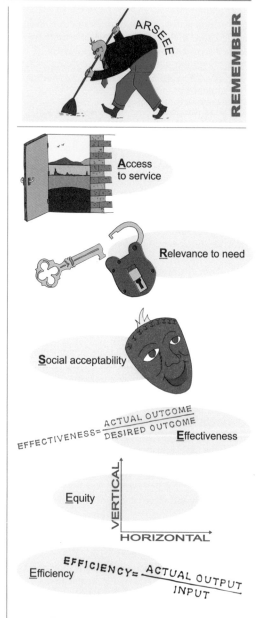

HEALTH CARE QUALITY

Maxwell's Criteria For Assessing Quality

Maxwell formulated a definition of health care quality which identified 6 different aspects (Maxwell, 1984):

Accessibility: This is concerned with the ease of availability/accessibility of services as and when they are required. Factors that impact upon access include:

- *Location barriers:* How far is the nearest dental practice?
- *Physical barriers:* Are there any stairs at the dental practice?
- *Availability:* What facilities (structure) and services (process) are there?
- *Organisational access:* What is the waiting time for appointments? Do they cater for language barriers? Is access to secondary care easy?
- *Financial costs of access:* Can the patient afford the transport, childcare or loss of earnings to come for an appointment?
- *Patient satisfaction:* Did the patient find the access acceptable?

Relevance to need: Relevance is centred on catering for the needs of the whole community by balancing the range of services offered.

Social acceptability: Treatments must be humane and services must conform to socially acceptable standards.

Effectiveness: Effectiveness is a measure of actual outcome compared to the desired outcome. The technical quality of treatment must be effective when individuals receive it. Often coordination and integration between professionals within organisations and between organisations impact beneficially upon health and quality of life of the individual. It is now widely accepted that the use of evidence-based practice will make care most effective.

Equity: Equity is defined as the extent to which all individuals in a population access the care they need. Equity can be classified as:

- *Horizontal equity:* Equally accessible effective care for all users so that persons with equal need receive the same level of health care.
- *Vertical equity:* Greater access to effective care for those with more need, so that greater need for services is met by greater use.

Efficiency: Efficiency is a measure of the ratio of actual output to given input.

REMEMBER

Access to service

Relevance to need

Social acceptability

$$EFFECTIVENESS = \frac{ACTUAL\ OUTCOME}{DESIRED\ OUTCOME}$$ Effectiveness

Equity

VERTICAL

HORIZONTAL

$$EFFICIENCY = \frac{ACTUAL\ OUTPUT}{INPUT}$$ Efficiency

Remember: For good quality, do not be **ARSE-EE**, remember Maxwell's criteria!

HEALTH CARE QUALITY (3)

Importance Of Quality Issues In Health Care

Quality issues in health care are more important now than ever before due to the following reasons:

- **I**atrogenesis incidence increased
- **M**arket philosophy
- **P**rofessional development
- **O**lder population
- **R**esource constraints and rising costs
- **T**echnology: Advances in medical technology
- **C**linical practice: Variations in clinical practice
- **E**ducated and better informed population

 Remember: **IMPORTanCE** of quality issues in health care

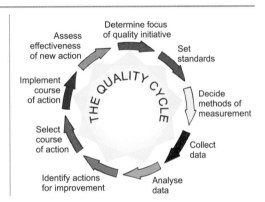

The Quality Cycle

The quality cycle is a process used to improve quality. Here it is shown as a 9-step cycle. The first step is to outline an aim for a quality initiative, followed by setting appropriate standards. The standards set should be SMART (see Chapter 3: Health Education). The methods of measurement are then decided and data are collected and analysed. This identifies actions for improvement. The penultimate stages of the cycle involve selecting and implementing an appropriate course of action. The final step involves assessing the effectiveness of the new action. The cyclic process can begin again with ever improving health care quality.

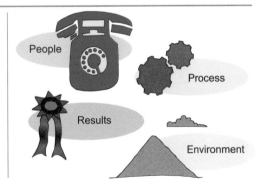

Health Quality Service

As described above the concepts of health care quality are both diverse and complex. The Health Quality Service has adopted a developmental approach to improving health care quality, the heart of which focuses on 4 key areas (examples given below):

- **People:** Better communication between staff and patients
- **Process:** Review all departmental practices
- **Environment:** Infection control surveillance system put in place
- **Results:** Better implementation of best practice

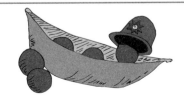

Achieving And Managing Quality

The techniques and tools for achieving and managing quality are listed below:

- **P**rofessional standard systems
- **O**utcome appraisal techniques
- **L**ocal problem identification techniques
- **I**nvolvement of consumer techniques
- **C**ase selection techniques
- **E**vidence: Record techniques
- **P**rocess appraisal techniques

 Remember: **Pea POLICE** patrol to achieve and manage quality!

CLINICAL GOVERNANCE

Definition

The concept of clinical governance was introduced in the White Paper 'Designed to Care'. The intention of the paper was that clinical governance would build on (not replace) existing patterns of self-regulation. The principles of clinical governance extend these procedures more widely and systematically into the local clinical community. It is a framework designed to improve the quality of health care by: identifying ways to improve quality, recognising and managing risk and ensuring continuing professional development.

A first class service: 'A framework through which NHS organisations are accountable for continuously improving the quality of their services and safeguarding high standards of care, by creating an environment in which excellence in clinical care will flourish'

NHSE, 1998

The 8 Building Blocks Of Clinical Governance

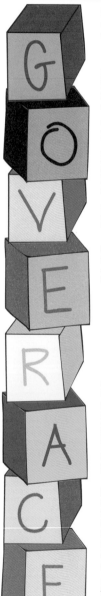

Greatest Health Care Practice (Implementation of Best Practice):
- Following the NICE guidelines e.g. extraction of wisdom teeth, frequency of recall
- RCS faculty of GDPs have information on many topics for implementation of best practice, including clinical examination, record keeping, adult antimicrobial prescribing, oral maxillofacial surgery, orthodontics, paediatric dentistry, restorative dentistry, and so on.

Openness and Accountability: Clinical governance belongs to the whole team. A lead is required who is in charge of clinical governance and accountable for its operation. It is very important to have a supportive environment with openness to change and there should be a quality policy which is accessible to patients.

Very Happy Patients (Patient Satisfaction): Use of patient surveys, suggestion/complaints box, user friendly treatment plans and information leaflets.

Every Year: Monitoring and Feedback: A comprehensive programme of activity which improves quality should be a regular occurrence. Baseline assessments should be recorded and a clinical improvement plan devised. The plan could include: practice developments and problems, complaints and incidents, training needs, audit activity, user strategy, and clinical effectiveness.

Risk Management: Some key topics for risk management would include: significant event audit, incident reporting, complaints, cross infection, and health and safety.

Audit and Peer Review: Clinical audit is simply a method of systematically checking the quality of a health service given to patients. It consists of the audit cycle and the audit project plan.
Audit Cycle: The audit cycle consists of a number of stages; it is a cyclical process aiming to achieve a positive change:

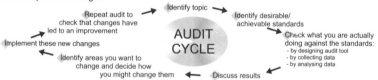

Audit Plan: The audit plan consists of a brief outline of the aims and objectives as well as the standards to be set. A summary of methodology, including details of data sample sizes, recording methods and proposed methods of data analysis are then noted. It is then followed by a timetable of activity with proposed educational source materials, and named facilitators and details of necessary meetings.
Peer review: Peer review is a method of sharing knowledge between colleagues with the aim of identifying areas in which changes can be made with the objective of improving the quality of service offered to patients. It is well structured with clearly defined goals. It is known to be of potential benefit for GDS patients.

Continuing Professional Development: All dentists on the Dentists' Register must undertake CPD for recertification every 5 years. The requirements are 250 hours over a 5 year period of which 75 hours are verifiable. Verifiable CPD includes courses organised by postgraduate dental deaneries, professional or scientific organisations, clinical audit and peer review, vocational training or general professional training study days, commercially run courses and long distance learning, incorporating as verifiable components and verifiable courses. All these courses require clear educational aims, objectives, anticipated outcomes and means of quality control. The course should also provide a certificate stating the title, dentist's name and number of verifiable hours.

Excellent Professional Performance: Healthcare provided should be based on evidence (evidence-based dentistry). Poor performance should be identified, reflected upon and improved through personal development plans and CPD. Staff appraisals should also be carried out frequently.

 Remember: **GOVERnAnCE** (ignore the n)

OPTIONS FOR CHANGE

Introduction

The two main problems with the 1990 NHS contract were the professional treadmill and patients finding no access to NHS dentistry. In September 2000, 'Modernising NHS Dentistry' focused on improving access, quality of dental care and oral health care.

The government is determined to bring dentistry back into the mainstream of the NHS and looks forward to working with the profession to make "Options for Change" a reality'.
David Lammy, August 2002
MP Parliamentary under Secretary of State for Health

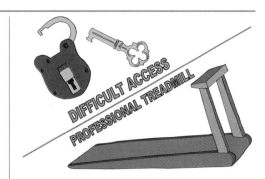

The 8 Themes

The 'Options for Change' strategy examined 8 themes in 28 field sites. The aim was to change the future of primary dental care. This was the biggest change facing dentists since 1948, with the fundamental change being in the organisation of payment and contracting General Dental Services (GDS) and new ways of delivering dentistry to the public.

1. **Local Commissioning and Funding**
- To secure access to high quality NHS dental service and improve oral health
- Devolved funding to PCTs for dentistry

2. **Methods of Remunerating General Dental Practitioners**
- Quality rather than quantity, options to be explored and tested

3. **Prevention and Oral Health Assessments for Patients**
- Proposal for a standard oral health assessment including prevention, lifestyle analysis and discussion of treatment options
- Individual timings on frequency of assessments ('check ups')

4. **Clinical Pathways**
- Appropriate and evidence-based treatment for patients based on agreed, evidence-based protocols

5. **Information and Communication Technology**
- Better use of ICT assisting clinical pathway approach, communication with patients and clinical governance

6. **Practice Structure**
- Anticipation of larger practices in the future encompassing improved skill mix

7. **Development of the Dental Team**
- Education, training and development of all members of the dental team

8. **Patient Experience**
- A new deal for patients with national standards. The priorities include access, receiving quality care, better information and oral health promotion

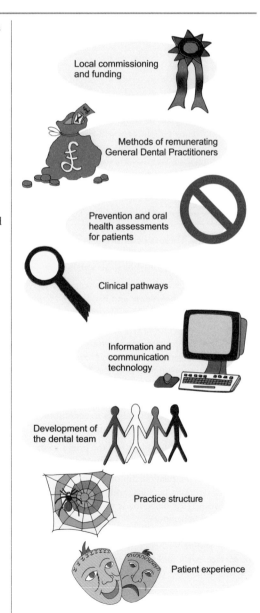

Local commissioning and funding

Methods of remunerating General Dental Practitioners

Prevention and oral health assessments for patients

Clinical pathways

Information and communication technology

Development of the dental team

Practice structure

Patient experience

BARRIERS TO ACCESS (1)

Definition

Access is concerned with the ease of availability/ accessibility of services as and when they are required. *Facilitating access* is concerned with helping people to command appropriate health care resources in order to preserve or improve their health:

- Is there an adequate supply?
- Are services affordable, accessible and acceptable?
- Are services relevant and effective?
- Are there differing perspectives and needs in diverse groups?

Why Bother?

The common problems with health care delivery are numerous. They include unequal distribution, lack of resources, inadequate emphasis on prevention, unclear goals, inadequate organisation, poor use of team dentistry, the payment methods and the lack of public accountability.

Understanding access to services is important (especially because of government policy) so that appropriate improvements can be made. For example, financial planning can be sought effectively after finding how many people were actually making regular use of dental services and what were the reasons behind non-use of services. Person-power planning can also be solved by providing supply where there is demand.

Penchansky And Thomas - The 5 A's (1981)

Penchasky and Thomas described barriers to access in terms of the 5 A's (Availability, Accessibility, Accommodation, Affordability, Acceptability):

Availability is the relationship of the volume and type of services to client volume and needs (e.g. How well are services distributed? Does limited perception of availability impact on uptake of care?).

Accessibility is the relationship between the location of supply and location of clients (e.g. How far do you travel to the nearest dental practice? What floor is the surgery on?).

Accommodation is the manner in which supply is organised related to clients' ability to accommodate to these factors (e.g. opening hours, drop in-centres).

Affordability is the relationship of the prices to the clients' income (e.g. direct and indirect costs).

Acceptability is the relationship of clients' attitudes regarding desirable personal and practice characteristics (e.g. being made to feel welcome, professional behaviour).

Note the difference between 'having access', which is the service exists, and 'gaining access', which is either entering or utilising the service.

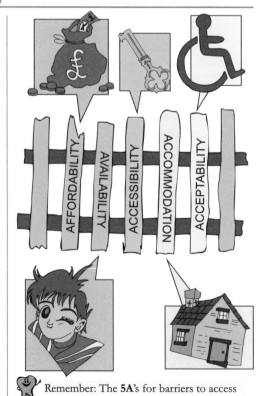

Remember: The **5A's** for barriers to access

BARRIERS TO ACCESS (2)

The Evidence For Barriers To Access

Many studies have reported barriers to access for different reasons. Bauer and Pierson in 1978 explained the service use by using 5 groups of variables: epidemiological, demographic, socio-economic, personal and psychological, and the characteristics of the system.

1. **Age and Gender:** The very old and very young rarely use dental services, with the peak usage being between 6 and 24 years. This is due to the natural history of disease, age and its relationship to social development, age related eligibility for free dental services and cohort changes. Women were found to use dental services more frequently than men, and they were more likely to be regular attenders. The reasons were because women attended with children and again the eligibility for free treatment during and after pregnancy.

2. **Socio-economic Status:** This is not a straightforward relationship. There was no difference in perceived importance of regular attendance between socio-economic groups.

3. **Ethnic Origin:** A larger proportion of whites than non-whites use the general dental services. The reasons for this were that there is a differing perception of need and the problem of language barrier.

4. **Perception of Need for Dental Care:** The value individuals put on health. Lower social classes place a lower value on preserving their teeth, they tend to opt for extraction as opposed to restoration. Self-assessment of dental health, attitudes and practices also vary among differing groups of people.

5. **Barriers to Attendance:** There are many factors that affect an individual's attendance at the dentist. All these factors act synergistically, hence it is important to tackle all these aspects and not just one:

- *Availability and Access:* in areas of low dentist to patient ratio there are longer waiting times and greater distances to travel. The community have to work harder and spend more to visit a dentist. Costs would include transport, telephone, time off work and child-care facilities.
- *Fear and Anxiety:* this is the next most common international barrier. Exacerbating these factors would include bad experience in the past and prolonged waiting time before examination.
- The *Internal Environment of the Practice:* influences on judgements of 'friendliness' include: seating arrangements, ceiling angle (sloped angles are more friendly than straight angles) and window shape (bow windows are more friendly than square ones).

In 1988, Finch found the following barriers to access: fear and cost of dental treatment, reception/waiting room procedures, loss of control, personality of the dentist, sounds, smells and white coats.

'They see you as a mouth'

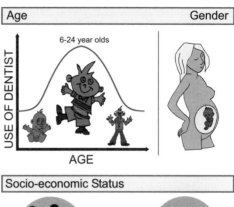

Age / Gender

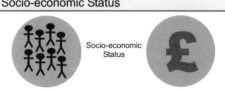

Socio-economic Status

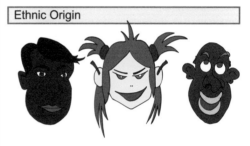

Ethnic Origin

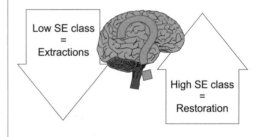

Perception of Need for Dental Care

Low SE class = Extractions

High SE class = Restoration

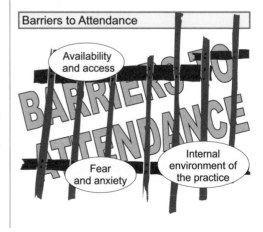

Barriers to Attendance

Availability and access

Fear and anxiety

Internal environment of the practice

BARRIERS TO ACCESS (3)

Adult Oral Health Survey

A National Survey carried out in 1998 confirmed the role of barriers and their impact upon attendance and treatment experience.

The National Survey set out 15 statements in total. Five statements were on aspects of fear, five were on aspects of dental practice organisation and the remaining five were related to costs of treatment. The national sample included 3,500 adults. These were the results obtained:

- 11% reported no barriers to dental care
- 45% selected a barrier related to fear
- 22% selected a barrier related to practice organisation/image
- 22% selected a barrier related to cost

It was also found that women were more likely to identify with statements than men, especially with regard to fear. Also, those individuals attending only when in trouble were more likely to associate themselves with all the statements, with fear as the most important. And finally, those individuals selecting a fear statement as most important had more missing teeth and fewer filled teeth, but similar numbers of sound and untreated teeth.

Barriers to Dental Care

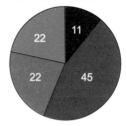

22	11
22	45

■ No barriers to dental care ■ Barrier related to fear
■ Barrier related to practice ■ Barrier related to cost

> women were more likely to identify with statements than men

> those individuals attending only when in trouble were more likely to associate themselves with all the statements

> those individuals selecting a fear statement as most important had more missing teeth and fewer filled teeth

At-Risk Groups

Disadvantage Group	Main problem	Additional problem	Possible solution
Learning difficulties	Communication	Other anxious people	Educate reception staff. Advocacy skills in carers
Physical disability	Mobility/stairs	Specialised transport	Identify practices with ground-floor access
Elderly housebound	Cannot leave house	Anxiety	Provide a domiciliary service
Lone low income parents	Childcare costs	Additional costs	Identify dentists who welcome children in waiting room

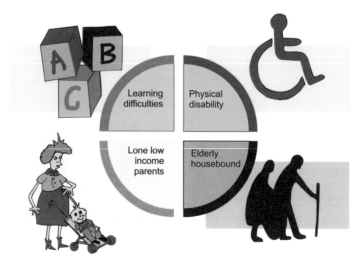

BARRIERS TO ACCESS (4)

Reducing The Barriers

Having understood the barriers to access it is important to act upon these and take appropriate measures to reduce them. Appropriate tools to improve access are health education and health promotion (Chapter 3). To summarise the key points:

Health Education involves:

- *Personal education and development* involve better communication, provide explanations and being friendly
- *Mass media information and education* involve advertising and raising awareness

Health Promotion involves:

- *Personal/preventive services* involve, reducing pain by making techniques more comfortable and emphasising the importance of prevention
- *Environmental measures* involve providing a better practice environment
- *Community development* to develop the lay assessment of need, self-help groups for anxiety and pressure groups to extend availability of services
- *Organisational change*, examples include continuing education for staff, changing hours of opening, employ advocates and practice leaflets
- *Economic and regulatory activities* such as free check-ups, displaying prices and free initial course of treatment

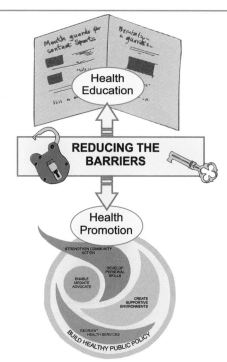

Health Promotion Logo adapted from WHO, 1986.
Adapted and reproduced with permission (see Permissions).

The Dudley Experiment

The Dudley experiment focused on 'improving supply and increasing demand'.

- **Improving Supply:** was to institute a programme of professional development which would help practitioners become aware of, and respond to the barriers to dental care as perceived by clients.
- **Increasing Demand:** was to test the use of generic advertising to try to overcome some of the perceived barriers to dental care, and to increase the uptake of general dental practitioner dental services by those people who did not attend regularly.

	Improving Supply	Increasing Demand
Method	• May 1989 - March 1990 • 8 workshops for dentists and staff • 38 practices, 95 dentists *Topics included:* • Marketing and dentistry • Giving patients information • Practice development • Barriers in GDP • Leading the dental team • Staff and patient surveys	• 'Dental update' for those not attending regularly. An invitation to approach a dental practice and discuss aspects of dental treatment • 'Generic' advertising: bus shelters, buses, household leaflets
Evaluation	• 1 or more practitioners from 19 practices attended 4+ workshops • 2 practices attended all workshops • 2 practices did not attend any • Attitudes of dentists (40 interviews): 16 ambivalent about marketing, 10 positive, 14 negative • 10 practices made 15 changes (leaflets, reminder system, more toys) *Barriers to professional development identified:* • No financial incentive • Will courses sustain practice development? • Limited confidence/time/expectations to introduce change • No need to change	• 44 people signed dental update attendance books • 18 out of 1000 people reported visiting a dentist, who had not attended in the previous two years (=600/month, approx. 15/practice) • 25% of a sample interviewed remembered some advertising/information related to dental issues, compared to 9% of the control group *The following was perceived by dentists:* • Encouraging non-attenders to become regular attenders • Not improving dental experience for patients • Having no impact on changing views or attendance • The 'new' patients were 'irregular attenders' rather than 'non-attenders'

THE ROADSIDE DENTIST (1)

In places where a formal health care system is not available, a different approach to dental care can be found. Our elective in rural India describes one such system. We observed the practice of an unqualified dentist working at the roadside - 'the roadside dentist'. Although this informal health care arrangement is available in many developing countries, they co-exist alongside more formal systems. This is not examinable material but helps one appreciate a health care system very different to one in a developed country.

Bridging The Service Gap

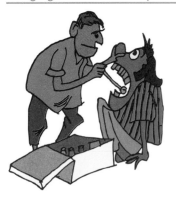

India has the largest number of dental schools in the world, almost 200 schools which produce around 12,000 newly qualified practitioners each year. Yet, despite the vast number of dentists, there are still too few qualified dental practitioners to provide an adequate service to India's one billion population - with just one dentist to every 40,000 inhabitants.

One often overlooked and largely undervalued source of dental treatment is the unqualified roadside dentist. His basic appliances include a folding chair, protective awning, bowl of water, rudimentary instruments and traditional post-operative potions. Countless thousands of such roadside dentists provide a readily accessible and affordable peripatetic service to their patients, who are among some of the poorest and most deprived members of the community.

Although Indian dentistry is as sophisticated as any in the world, extraction remains the most common form of treatment amongst the illiterate poor. Since the services of a qualified practitioner are not easily accessible to the vast majority of the population, the gap is filled literally at the roadside by the ubiquitous unqualified practitioner. This affordable service is largely extraction based and available without appointment.

Profile Of The Roadside Dentist

Kesavbhai G Patel is in his fifties and an agricultural farmer by caste. Sent away by his father at the age of 15 to train under an experienced roadside practitioner in Mumbai, he returned to Gujarat at 18 to begin his practice.

With no formal qualification, he believes it is his duty to utilise his talent to assist the poorer members of society.

The Location

He practises in the southern part of Gujarat State, close to Mumbai on the west coast of India. His work extends over four towns located in three districts with a combined population of some 5 million (red circles on the diagram below).

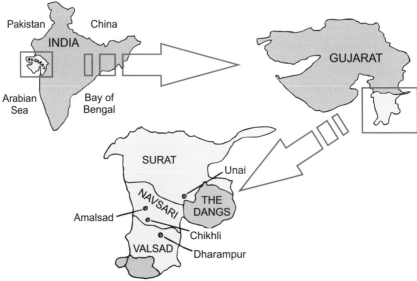

THE ROADSIDE DENTIST (2)

The Dental Surgery

His surgery is limited in both premises and equipment. He stands to treat his patients, who sit on a folding chair. A simple awning protects them from the scorching sun and monsoon rain. A bowl of dettol-infused water is used for disinfecting instruments. A bucket of cold water and steel cup are used for hand-washing and mouth-rinsing.

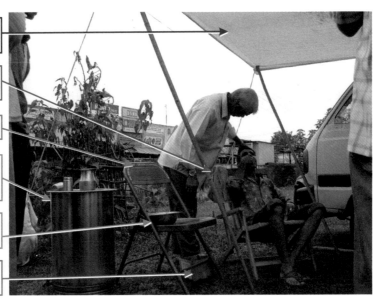

Tent provides shade and protects against the monsoon rains

Towel used to dry hands and also placed on patient's head

Fold-up **chair** for patient to sit on

Large bucket of **water** and steel cup for rinsing mouth after extraction and to wash hands

Bowl of dettol-infused water for **disinfection** of instruments

Clinical waste bin (cardboard box) for extracted teeth

Patient Management

History and Examination

Patients turn up at the roadside clinic without appointment. On payment of a flat rate, 20 rupees (approx. £0.30) patients collect a token and wait their turn. The roadside dentist asks each patient what is wrong and to indicate the affected tooth with their finger. He then examines the troublesome tooth with his fingers and gives his opinion on the need for extraction. (Note: He will extract anything up to 32 teeth in a single appointment for 20 rupees.)

Digital Anaesthesia

With the patient seated in the folding chair, the roadside dentist uses pressure from his fingers and/or thumb around the extraction site without using local anaesthesia. Further pressure is applied to the area following extraction. The area is subsequently rubbed vigorously. Finally, the patient is asked to stand up and spit out any saliva or blood from their mouth onto the ground.
'Getting a firm grip and being as quick as possible is how I extract painlessly without local anaesthetic.' Kesavbhai Patel

Post-operative Treatment

Following treatment, the patient is given a teaspoon of a home-made black powder to hold over the extraction site for around 10 minutes and then told to rinse with water. This is believed to alleviate pain and achieve haemostasis. In the infrequent case that bleeding continues, a secondary backup home-made potion is applied over the extraction site.

Complications and Referral

Of the 50 patients studied, only two had complications (fractured teeth). After trying unsuccessfully to remove the roots, the roadside dentist discharged the patients and told them to return if they were in pain.

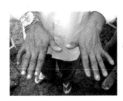

'The Healing Hands'

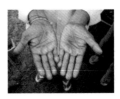

THE ROADSIDE DENTIST (3)

Patient Management: Photo Story

The photos below depict the actions taken by the roadside dentist on a typical visit.

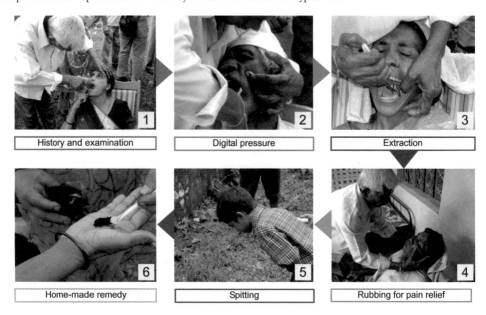

1 History and examination	**2** Digital pressure	**3** Extraction
6 Home-made remedy	**5** Spitting	**4** Rubbing for pain relief

Consent And Litigation

Informed consent is not obtained from the patient. The roadside dentist simply confirms in each case the tooth in question. If the patient agrees, extraction takes place, with no further explanation or warning. Where adjacent teeth are affected, these too are extracted if the patient agrees. Neither the Bolam Principle nor the Prudent Patient Standard applies, and litigation is not an issue. Patients consider themselves lucky to be free from pain at minimal cost. Post-operative complications such as swelling, pain or fractures are generally accepted.

Patient-Dentist Relationship

Patients respect the roadside dentist enormously. Some believe he has special powers from God and a few female patients tie a rakhi (string bracelet) on his wrist, symbolising a brother-sister relationship. Most of his patients are reluctant to visit the hospital or dental clinic for reasons of social class, status or language barriers. They visit him because they feel comfortable discussing their problems with a 'local man', who they feel is one of them, more understanding and less intimidating.

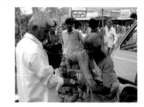

Health And Safety

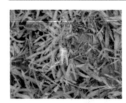

The clinic has no safe method for disposing of clinical waste. He gathers all the extracted teeth in a cardboard box, which he disposes of at any roadside rubbish pile at the end of each working day.

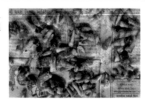

THE ROADSIDE DENTIST (4)

Patient Experience

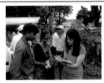

The roadside dentist saw 322 patients in the five days we spent with him - over 60 each day. We carried out a structured interview on 50 patients chosen at random, in Gujarati (the native language).

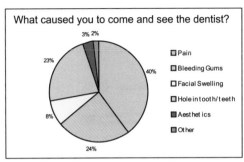

What caused you to come and see the dentist?

- Pain
- Bleeding Gums
- Facial Swelling
- Hole in tooth/teeth
- Aesthetics
- Other

Cause of visit

Most (40%) visited the roadside dentist because they experienced pain. Bleeding gums (24%), a hole in their tooth (23%) and facial swelling (8%) were the next most common causes. Aesthetics was not a common presenting complaint. Almost three-quarters (72%) of the patients knew of an alternative source of dental practice such as a conventional dentist. Travel, treatment cost and social class were the main factors limiting access to conventional dentists.

Visit regularity

Patients appear to suffer dental disease in silence, reporting for treatment only when the pain becomes intolerable. Two-thirds felt there was no benefit from visiting regularly. Most (94%) patients were manual workers, and at least half were illiterate. These factors may have influenced the frequency of visits. For most, this was their first visit, although one patient had visited four times previously. The roadside dentist sees new patients every day, most of whom have heard of him only by word of mouth, his only form of advertising.

Treatment satisfaction

Most (94%) patients were satisfied with their treatment. Sixty percent reported experiencing mild or no pain and a further 20% only average pain. Reasons for this level of satisfaction and apparent lack of pain could be many. Factors could range from removal of intolerable toothache at minimum cost to a belief in the dentist's God-given powers.

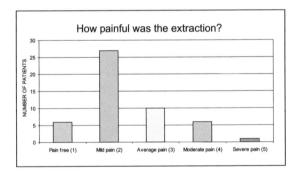

How painful was the extraction?

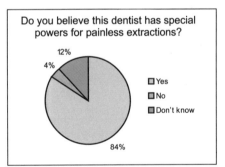

Do you believe this dentist has special powers for painless extractions?

- Yes
- No
- Don't know

12%
4%
84%

Cross-infection

The roadside dentist does not wear gloves, mask or protective eye-wear. Although no one interviewed knew what cross-infection was, 4% thought its control was unimportant, 38% did not think the dentist was carrying it out and 62% were unsure whether he was. He rinses his hands in water without disinfectant between patients. His only form of instrument sterilisation was to keep them in a bowl of cold dettol-infused water in between use.

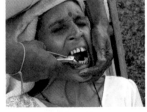

Bloody hands and instruments

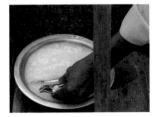

Instruments rinsed in dettol-infused water

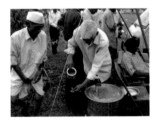

Hands rinsed in water without disinfectant

THE ROADSIDE DENTIST (5)

Patient Experience (continued)

Oral hygiene

Approximately two-thirds (68%) of patients clean their teeth once daily and 30% twice daily. Forty-two percent clean their teeth using a brush, 35% using daatun sticks and 19% using their finger. Many brands of toothpaste are available in India, from commercially available brands to ayurvedic powder brands. Daatun are 10-inch sticks of fresh, undried tree branches, far cheaper than brush and toothpaste. The stick is chewed from end to end. The chewed fibres are later used as a tongue scraper. The table illustrates some types of daatun with their believed function:

Daatun		Colour	Taste	Believed function
Baavad		Dark green	Astringent	Removes bad odour
Limdo		Brown	Very bitter	Anti-bacterial
Karanj		Grey/ pale green	Bitter	Anti-bacterial
Vaad		Light brown	Sweet	Teeth-whitening

Abusive habits

Betel, paan and guthka (tobacco) chewing is socially acceptable and widespread in India, with 60% to 70% of my sample admitting to all three. The cheap, appetite-depressing guthka packages are particularly popular among street children, as well as adults, who can go through up to 15 packets a day. This is causing concern amongst dentists and doctors, since it can give rise to cancerous lesions in the mouth and a long-term chewing habit can lead to severe attrition, abrasion and gingival recession.

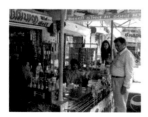
Street vendors selling paan and guthka

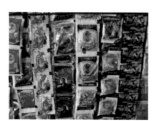
Guthka packets

Better Than Nothing

While all is not quite as it should be, with little in the way of formal qualification, infection control, or health and safety precautions the roadside dentist with his basic tools continues to fulfil a popular and indispensable role in the community, relieving masses of deprived members from pain.

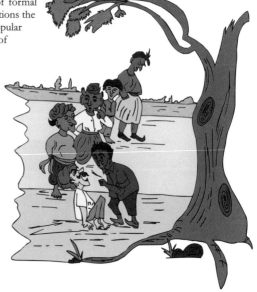

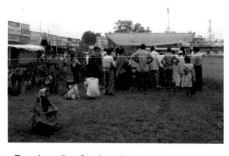
People gather for dental treatment every day

QUESTIONS

Short Answer Questions

1. Briefly describe three key strengths of the National Health Service (NHS). Provide a dental example to illustrate two of these points. (3 marks)
2. There are a number of ways dentists can be paid. List them and list the advantages and disadvantages of each payment method you have listed. (2 marks)
3. Three dimensions of access are availability, accommodation and accessibility. List and define the other two. (2 marks)
4. Choose any two of the access dimensions. For each dimension propose one way of reducing the barriers it creates. (2 marks)
5. Social and economic factors are two of four major groups of environmental factors that influence the organisation and delivery of oral health care. List the other two. (1 mark)
6. Name one socio-demographic and one attitudinal trend which may impact on the delivery of oral health care. (2 marks)
7. How might the socio-demographic trend you have named impact on the delivery of oral health care? (1 mark)
8. How might the attitudinal trend you have named impact on the delivery of oral health care? (1 mark)
9. What definition has been proposed for an oral health care system? (1 mark)
10. Political/legal and technological factors are two of four major groups of factors that influence the organisation and delivery of oral health care. List the other two. (1 mark)
11. Name one political/legal and one technological factor which may influence the organisation and delivery of oral health care. (2 marks)
12. How would you define 'health care quality'? (1 mark)
13. Maxwell has proposed six dimensions of health care quality. State four of them. (2 marks)
14. Give two reasons for the increasing interest in health care quality. (2 marks)
15. The General Dental Service (GDS) is the major source of NHS dental care. List the other sources of NHS dental care. (1 mark)

Long Answer Questions

Write short notes on the following topics. Up to 4 marks will be awarded for your answer.
1. The role of the UK Community Dental Service (CDS).
2. The key components of a health care system.
3. The possible advantages and disadvantages for oral health with regard to the main methods of paying dental workers.
4. Patient and professional views about quality and the implications of these for quality assurance programmes in general dental practice.
5. The advantages and disadvantages of capitation and fee-for-item payment methods.
6. Lay and professional views about quality and the implications for general dental practice.
7. The different methods of funding oral health care systems.
8. The concept of access applied to dental care.
9. The meaning of General Professional Training (GPT) and its opportunities for the dental profession.
10. Barriers to seeking dental care.
11. The reasons for and proposed requirements of the GDC's re-certification programme.
12. Vocational Training (VT) and the benefits it should bring for new graduates.
13. The main content and conclusions of the Dudley study to increase the uptake of primary dental care.

Essay Questions

You will be awarded up to 20 marks for your answer.
1. What do you understand by the term 'access'. Outline the policy proposals you would make to improve access to primary dental care, giving reasons for your choice of proposals.
2. Outline the four key messages for the prevention of dental diseases and the scientific background of these messages.

MY NOTES AND SPIDERGRAM

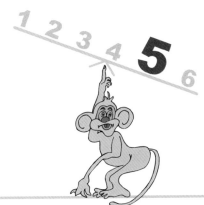

Preventive Dentistry

CHAPTER 5

5

AIMS AND OBJECTIVES

Introduction To Preventive Strategies

Aim

To introduce different preventive strategies for disease prevention

Objectives
- Define strategy
- Understand the general principles in developing an oral health promotion strategy
- Discuss the features of a population, high-risk and targeted population strategy

Introduction To Screening

Aim

To understand the general principles of screening

Objectives
- Define screening, mass screening and population screening
- Understand the difference between screening and diagnosis
- List and understand the general principles of screening
- Discuss the validation of screening for oral diseases

Preventive Strategies: Dental Caries

Aim

To understand the strategies used for the prevention of dental caries

Objectives
- List the factors associated with dental caries
- Apply the general principles of preventive strategies to dental caries

Preventive Strategies: Periodontal Diseases

Aim

To understand the strategies used for the prevention of periodontal diseases

Objectives
- List the factors associated with periodontal diseases
- Apply the general principles of preventive strategies to periodontal diseases

Preventive Strategies: Oral Cancer

Aim

To understand the strategies used for the prevention of oral cancer

Objectives
- Describe the distribution of oral cancer in terms of gender and geography
- Outline the key aetiological factors for oral cancer
- Describe possible health promotion strategies required to prevent oral cancer

Smoking Cessation

Aim

To understand the concepts underlying smoking cessation

Objectives
- To explain current trends in tobacco use
- To list the oral health impacts of tobacco use
- To outline the potential role of the primary dental care practice team in tobacco cessation
- To review issues associated with tobacco use: starting, quitting, dependency, general health risks and withdrawal symptoms
- To describe the role of primary dental care in tobacco cessation

INTRODUCTION TO PREVENTIVE STRATEGIES

Definition

A *strategy* is defined as a broad plan of action which specifies what is to be achieved and how to achieve it, and which provides a framework for more detailed planning.

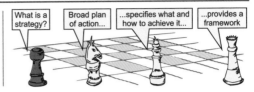

Developing An Oral Health Promotion Strategy

Developing an oral health promotion strategy comprises a cyclical process. One must consider the following three questions:

What are you trying to achieve?
- Identify needs and priorities
- Setting clear aims and objectives
- Objectives must be 'SMART' (see Chapter 3: Health Education for details)

What are you going to do?
- Identify possible methods of achieving your aims and objectives
- Selecting the best methods
- Identifying resources to be used
- Setting a clear action plan of who does what and when

How would you know whether or not you have been successful?
- Develop methods of process evaluation
- Develop methods of outcome evaluation

1. Identify needs and priorities

2. Set clear aims and objectives

3. Decide the best way of achieving the aim

4. Identify resources

5. Set an action plan

6. Plan evaluation methods

Preventive Strategies

In the widest context, preventive dentistry covers all aspects of dentistry and includes those practices by individuals and communities that affect oral health status. There are three main prevention methods:
- **Primary prevention** centres on preventing disease initiation by the use of health promotion, health education and the common risk factor approach.
- **Secondary prevention** involves impeding disease progression and recurrence through early diagnosis and treatment for those who have disease.
- **Tertiary prevention** focuses on replacement methods such as providing services to stop the loss of function through rehabilitation.

An oral health promotion strategy focuses more towards a social model. To change from dental orientation to lay competence, from authoritarian health education to supportive health education and from individualistic behaviour modification to a systemic population strategy using public health approaches.

Health Promotion Strategies

Health promotion can be targeted at specific groups of the population.
- **High-risk population strategy** focuses efforts on high-risk individuals, attempting to lower the level of risk factors at the unfavourable end of the distribution. This will shift the end of the distribution of exposure and disease in a favourable direction.
- **Whole population strategy** focuses efforts on the whole population. It attempts to lower the mean level of risk factors, to shift the whole distribution of exposure and disease in a favourable direction.
- **Targeted population strategy** focuses efforts on a targeted population. It attempts to lower the mean level of risk factors of a targeted population, to shift the whole distribution of exposure and disease of a targeted population in a favourable direction.

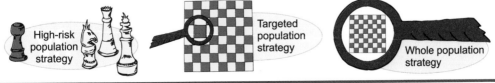

INTRODUCTION TO SCREENING

Definition

Dental screening is the presumptive identification of unrecognised disease or defect by the application of tests, examinations or other procedures, which can be applied rapidly (Commission on Chronic Illness, 1957). Screening tests are initiated by the medical professional rather than the patient, offering tests to individuals who are apparently healthy with the purpose of separating them into groups having high and low probability for a particular disorder. There is a moral obligation to inform individuals of the result of their screening test. If tested positive the patient should be referred for further diagnosis and treatment. A screening test should not be diagnostic.

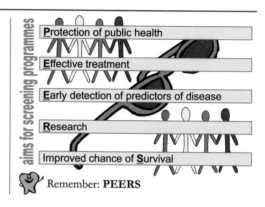

aims for screening programmes

- Protection of public health
- Effective treatment
- Early detection of predictors of disease
- Research
- Improved chance of Survival

Remember: **PEERS**

Types Of Screening

There are two main types of screening available, mass screening and selective screening. *Mass screening* involves screening on a large scale, as the name suggests; screening the whole population where no selection of population groups is made. In contrast, *selective screening* is aimed specifically at screening the high-risk groups.

Mass Screening
Large-scale screening without selection

Selective Screening
High-risk groups screening

Principles Of Screening

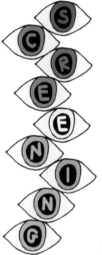

- **Suitable and acceptable test:** There should be a suitable test available
- **Cost:** The screening programme should be balanced against the benefit it provides
- **Repeat screening** at intervals for diseases of insidious onset, for diagnosis and treatment of abnormalities detected
- **Early recognisable stage:** There should be an early recognisable stage of the disease
- **Early stage treatment** of disease should be of more benefit than treatment started at a later stage
- **Natural history** of the disease should be well understood
- **Important health problem:** The condition sought should be an important health problem
- **provisioN for diagnosis and treatment:** There should be adequate facilities for the diagnosis and treatment of abnormalities detected
- **physioloGical** and physical harm to those screened should be less than the chance of benefit

 Remember: The principles of **SCREENING!**

Validation Of Screening

- **Sensitivity:** The ability of a test to give a positive finding when the person tested truly has the disease
- **Specificity:** The ability of a test to give a negative finding when the person tested is free of the disease under study
- **Positive Predictive Value:** The proportion of people with positive test results being correctly labelled diseased
- **Negative Predictive Value:** The proportion of people with negative test results being correctly labelled non-diseased

TRUE DISEASE STATUS OF INDIVIDUAL

		Affected (Disease)	Unaffected (No Disease)	
SCREENING TEST RESULT	Positive (Abnormal)	a True-positive	b False-positive	PPV
	Negative (Normal)	c False-negative	d True-negative	NPV
		Sensitivity	Specificity	

Specificity = d/(b+d)	PPV = a/(a+b)
Sensitivity = a/(a+c)	NPV = d/(c+d)

PREVENTIVE STRATEGIES: DENTAL CARIES (1)

Summary Of Trends

There are a number of factors associated with the decline in caries as discussed in Chapter 2. Here is a brief description of the trends and variations in caries experience.

There has been a remarkable, well documented decline in caries experience amongst children observed in most of the industrialised countries in recent decades. In this, the UK is no exception. Sources of data to describe the changes in the UK are the National Surveys (1973, 1983, 1993), BASCoD Surveys and occasional surveys (e.g. National Diet and Nutritional Survey). The caries criteria adopted is the 'into dentine' threshold. The data demonstrated the following:

In 5-year-olds from 1973-1983:
- dmft has decreased from 4.0 to 2.1
- Caries free increased from 30% to 50%

In 12-year-olds from 1973-1992:
- DMFT has decreased from 4.8 to 1.2

In 15-year-olds from 1973-1983-1993:
- DMFT has decreased from 8.4 to 5.9 to 2.5
- Caries free children had increased from 7% in 1983 to 37% in 1993
- Proportion with some filled teeth decreased from 85% to 52%

Summary Of Variations

The key variations in levels of caries in children are explained by social class (lower = worse) and geography (the North-South divide). Studies suggest that higher caries levels can be identified as one of a range of factors which impact adversely upon multiply deprived and disadvantaged communities (Gratrix and Holloway, 1994; Ellwood and O'Mullane, 1995).

The data also suggest there is a changing distribution from Gaussian ('normal') to bimodal, which has led to the articulation of the 80/20 rule (i.e. that 80% of caries can be found in 20% of the population).

Factors Associated With Caries Decline

The various factors that have led to a decline in dental caries are listed below:
- Use of fluorides is usually recognised as the best single explanation
- Greater availability of preventive oral health services
- Increased dental awareness
- Improving education, living and working conditions
- Less sucrose use in households
- Changes in caries diagnosis and measurement
- Changes in treatment philosophy

Sheiham (1984) suggested that there was no one single explanation, but a combination of factors.

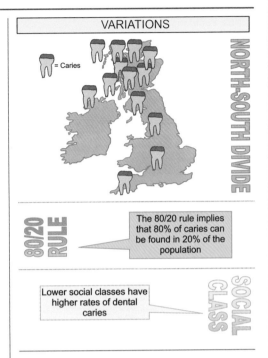

VARIATIONS

= Caries

NORTH-SOUTH DIVIDE

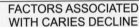

80/20 RULE

The 80/20 rule implies that 80% of caries can be found in 20% of the population

Lower social classes have higher rates of dental caries

SOCIAL CLASS

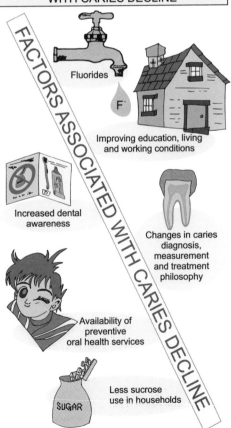

FACTORS ASSOCIATED WITH CARIES DECLINE

FACTORS ASSOCIATED WITH CARIES DECLINE

Fluorides

Improving education, living and working conditions

Increased dental awareness

Changes in caries diagnosis, measurement and treatment philosophy

Availability of preventive oral health services

Less sucrose use in households

SUGAR

PREVENTIVE STRATEGIES: DENTAL CARIES (2)

Primary Preventive Strategies

Whole Population Strategy

The prevalence of dental caries is low among adolescents, but high among adults. The main cause of dental caries is high sugar consumption, which is widespread in the population. The most effective way of preventing dental caries is the use of fluorides as it can be easily applied to the whole population (e.g. water fluoridation).

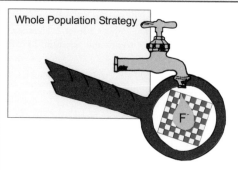
Whole Population Strategy

Targeted Population Strategy

A small group of adolescents have a high level of dental caries. Additional preventive programmes may be developed for those with high levels of dental caries (e.g. topical fluoride therapy which is applied by the patient at home or dental hygienists at school).

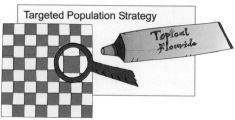
Targeted Population Strategy

Health Education and Health Promotion

To increase the awareness and knowledge of the benefits of eating healthily and the damaging effect of high sugar consumption, as well as the use of fluorides in caries prevention.

Use of fluoride has shown the following reductions:
1. Water fluoridation: 30-90%
2. Fluoride tablets: 40-80%
3. Fluoride dentifrice: 15-60%
4. Fluoride rinses: 30-40%
5. Fluoride gels: 23-33%

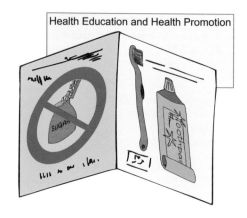
Health Education and Health Promotion

Common Risk Factor Approach

The main cause of dental caries is diet, which is also related to general health. Poor diet can result in obesity, diabetes, cancers and cardiovascular disease. Hence, targeting the idea of a good and healthy diet maximises resources by targeting the risk factor common to many conditions (see Chapter 3).

Secondary Preventive Strategies

To treat people known to have decay by applying measures to prevent physical, psychological and social disability, pain and tooth loss.

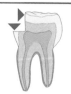

Treatment of disease

PREVENTIVE STRATEGIES: PERIODONTAL DISEASES

Public Health Aspects

Brief summary of the factors affecting the public health issues of periodontal diseases:

- Severe periodontitis is very rare
- Most adults exhibit some gingival inflammation or some loss of bone and probing attachment, but without pain, discomfort and loss of functioning dentition
- Tooth loss may occur, but only due to severe periodontitis
- Preventable and treatable at a population level?
- Very low financial cost

Summary of trends (see Chapter 2 for more detail):

- Proportion of dentate adults with periodontal pockets of 4mm or more increases with age
- Proportion of dentate adults with loss of attachment of 4mm or more also increases with age

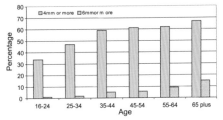

Proportion of dentate adults with periodontal pockets of 4mm or more by age in UK

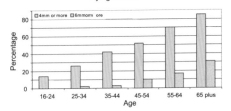

Proportion of dentate adults with loss of attachment of 4mm or more by age in UK

Primary Preventive Strategy

Whole Population Strategy: Mild periodontitis and gingivitis are almost universally prevalent. The known causes of periodontal diseases are bacterial dental plaque, tobacco smoking and psychosocial factors which are widespread in the population.

- A small reduction in the overall **plaque level** per year would reduce the general level of periodontal diseases, in particular gingivitis
- A small reduction in the number of **smokers** per year would reduce the general level of periodontal diseases, in particular periodontitis
- A small reduction in the overall level of **stress** per year would contribute to the reduction of plaque levels and the number of smokers, thus, the general level of periodontal diseases

Health Education and Health Promotion: To increase awareness and knowledge of good oral hygiene behaviour and the damaging effects of tobacco smoking and stress.

Common Risk Factor Approach: The known causes of periodontal diseases are hygiene, tobacco smoking and psychosocial factors, which are related to life-threatening diseases. Periodontal health education and promotion measures should be incorporated into general health policies (see Chapter 3).

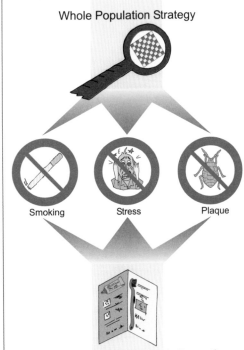

Whole Population Strategy

Smoking   Stress   Plaque

Health Education and Health Promotion

Secondary Preventive Strategy

- To treat people known to have severe periodontitis
- Applying measures to influence the course of detected disease and to reduce tooth loss

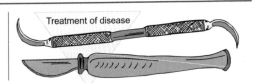

Treatment of disease

PREVENTIVE STRATEGIES: ORAL CANCER (1)

Introduction

Oral cancer is one of the few lethal diseases that dentists may encounter professionally. Every year in the UK, there are approximately 4,400 new cases, and 1,700 deaths. An annual incidence of around 7.5 per 100,000 with more males affected (Office for National Statistics, 2004).

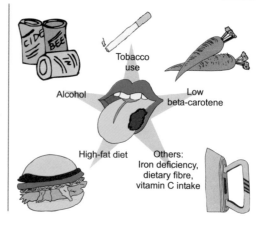

Tobacco use

Alcohol

Low beta-carotene

High-fat diet

Others: Iron deficiency, dietary fibre, vitamin C intake

Risk Factors

- Tobacco use (variation by type of use, type of tobacco and tar content)
- Alcohol consumption (synergistic effect)
- High-fat diet
- Low intake of beta-carotene
- Low dietary iron, fibre and vitamin C

Distribution Of Oral Cancer

Gender and Site: Registrations of newly diagnosed cases of oral cancer (UK, 2001):

Location	Men	Women
Lip	159	79
Tongue	627	364
Gum	106	88
Mouth	440	255
Palate	119	104

Region: Different regions in the world have varying social habits. For example:
- India: paan with tobacco is socially acceptable
- USA: 'snuff dipping' amongst baseball players

Area Based Survival: The affluent tend to be better educated and well-informed hence they are in better health. This population group are more likely to use health services and seek better quality care. In general, social deprivation is related to increased alcohol and tobacco use and poor nutrition.

Women tend to have better survival rates as they more readily act upon symptoms. In addition, women (the 'natural carers') take their children to the dentist and book appointments to be seen too.

Site and gender distributions of newly diagnosed cases

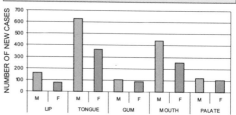

Regional differences

Paan   Snuff

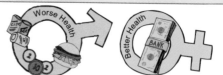

Area Based Survival

Age and gender distributions of newly diagnosed cases

Age and Gender: Registrations of newly diagnosed cases of oral cancer (UK, 2003):

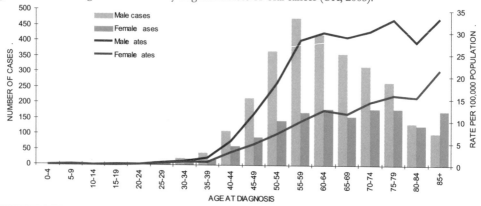

PREVENTIVE STRATEGIES: ORAL CANCER (2)

Oral Pre-cancer

Premalignant lesions have a low rate of transformation, 2-4% for leukoplakia and 1% for lichen planus. Premalignant lesions are usually asymptomatic and consist of the following features: colour (red speckling), texture (roughened surface), location (lateral border of the tongue, floor of the mouth, lower buccal sulcus).

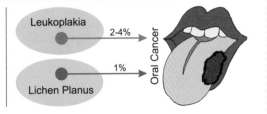

Health Promotion Strategy Using The Ottawa Charter Principles

Health promotion adopts a multi-factorial approach. There is a shift of responsibility from the health care system to individuals, communities and decision-makers at all levels of society. It involves developing a wider range of competencies to develop a complementary range of activities. The principles of the Ottawa Charter (described in Chapter 3) can be used to prevent oral cancer.

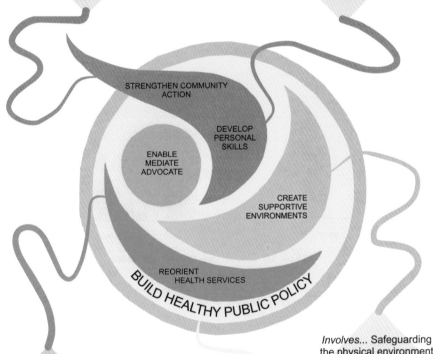

Involves... Health promotion through concrete and effective community work in setting priorities, making decisions, planning strategies and implementing them to prevent oral cancer.
(e.g. smoking cessation clinics)

Invloves... Personal and social education for healthier living.
(e.g. educating school children on the effects of smoking and alcohol)

STRENGTHEN COMMUNITY ACTION

DEVELOP PERSONAL SKILLS

ENABLE MEDIATE ADVOCATE

CREATE SUPPORTIVE ENVIRONMENTS

REORIENT HEALTH SERVICES

BUILD HEALTHY PUBLIC POLICY

Involves... Individuals, communities, health professionals, health services and governments to work together. There is a move towards preventing oral cancer, not just treating it.
(e.g. greater number of smoking cessation professionals)

Involves... Policy makers of all sectors and at all levels to take responsibility for health.
(e.g. greater constraints on tobacco and alcohol advertising)

Involves... Safeguarding the physical environment to help create a healthy society.
(e.g. no smoking areas)

Diagram adapted from WHO, 1986. Adapted and reproduced with permission (see Permissions).

PRACTICAL APPROACHES TO SMOKING CESSATION (1)

Who Smokes?

Twenty-eight percent of UK adults smoke. In 1996 it was seen that there was a distinct social class gradient, with 12% of professional men and 40% of unskilled manual workers smoking. Another at-risk group are young teenage women. Public health issues include:

- Smoking kills 120,000 people a year
- Treating smoking-related diseases costs the NHS up to £1.7 billion every year
- 17,000 children under 5 are admitted to hospital each year due to their parents smoking (Watt *et al.*, 2003)

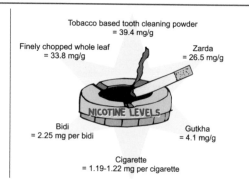

Tobacco based tooth cleaning powder = 39.4 mg/g

Finely chopped whole leaf = 33.8 mg/g

Zarda = 26.5 mg/g

NICOTINE LEVELS

Bidi = 2.25 mg per bidi

Gutkha = 4.1 mg/g

Cigarette = 1.19-1.22 mg per cigarette

Trends In Tobacco Use

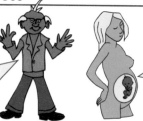

- In 1978 40% of 16+ smoked and in 1998 27%
- Social class: Higher prevalence in manual than non-manual
- 75% of lone parents
- 43% of men and 36% of women aged 20-24 years smoke

- 30% of women smoke during pregnancy
- 51% of young (16-24 years) pregnant women from manual social classes smoke

- 9% of 11-15 year olds smoke
- At 15 years, 28% of boys and 33% of girls

Estimates Of Individual Costs Of Smoking

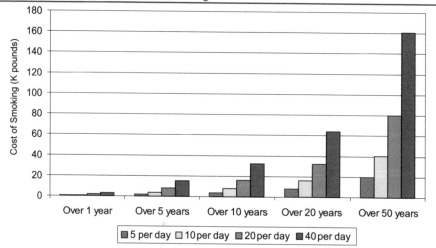

Cost of Smoking (K pounds)

■ 5 per day ☐ 10 per day ■ 20 per day ■ 40 per day

Oral Health Impacts Of Tobacco Use

Watt *et al.* (2003) reported 2,000 cases of oral cancer annually. There is a high mortality rate with 50% survival after 5 years. Tobacco users are 2-4 times more likely to suffer from oral cancer and 6 times more likely to have pre-maligant lesions such as leukoplakias compared to non-smokers.

Tobacco use is an independent risk factor for periodontal diseases, with a 2.5 to 6 fold rise. Wound healing is also adversely affected by tobacco use.

There are also social implications with the use of tobacco such as staining, changes in taste and halitosis. The palate can also become pigmented.

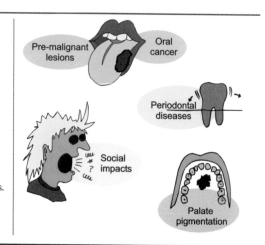

Pre-malignant lesions

Oral cancer

Periodontal diseases

Social impacts

Palate pigmentation

PRACTICAL APPROACHES TO SMOKING CESSATION (2)

Facilitating Smoking Cessation In Primary Dental Care

Smoking cessation can be facilitated in the primary dental care setting by:
- **I**ncentives
- **T**eam working
- **T**raining
- **I**mproved communication
- **M**ulti-disciplinary working
- **E**xamples of good practice
- **R**elevant resources

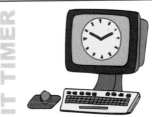

 Remember: **IT TIMER** for smoking cessation

The Change Model described by Prochaska and DiClemente in 1983 can be utilised to change patient behaviour. The stages are pre-contemplation, contemplation, preparation, action and maintenance. They are described in detail in Chapter 3.

Example:
How do you feel about stopping smoking?
- I have no desire to stop smoking and I do not intend to do so in the next six months
  (Pre-contemplation: The contented smoker)
- I have been smoking recently but I would like to consider stopping in the next six months
  (Contemplation: The concerned smoker)
- I have been smoking recently but I really want to stop in the next month *(Preparation)*
- I stopped smoking recently and I intend to carry on doing so in the next six months
  (Action/Maintenance: The contented ex-smoker)

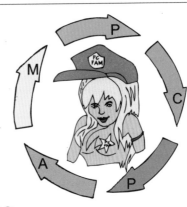

 Remember: **PC PAM**ela

Types Of Tobacco Cessation Service

Level 1: Very brief intervention provided in the normal course of professional duty
- 4 A's: ask, advise, assist and arrange
- 30 seconds-3 minutes
- 'Repetition reduces impact'

Level 2: Intermediate level intervention on a one-to-one basis by a trained adviser
- 4 A's (ask, advise, assist and arrange) and follow-up (NRT)
- 10-30 minutes

Level 3: Specialist tobacco cessation clinics

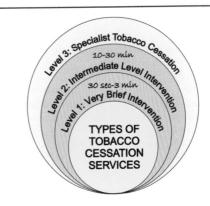

Smoking Cessation Guidelines For Health Professionals

The role of primary health care teams, hospitals and community trusts in tobacco cessation are as follows:

- Check status and keep records up to date
- Advise current smokers to stop (referral and record)
- Involve other primary care team members
- Smoke free environment
- Focus on the pregnant smoker
- Training for effectiveness

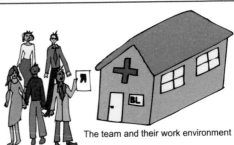

The team and their work environment

5

PRACTICAL APPROACHES TO SMOKING CESSATION (3)

Implementing The 4A's

Ask

- All patients should have their tobacco use status checked
- Update patient record

Tobacco smoking:
1. Do you have your first cigarette within 20 minutes of waking?
2. Do you smoke at least 10-20 cigarettes regularly each day?

Tobacco chewing:
1. Do you chew tobacco in your paan?
2. Do you have your first paan with tobacco within one hour of waking?

Advise

All smokers should be advised on the value of quitting:

- How do you feel about smoking/chewing?
- The best thing you can do for your general and oral health is to stop smoking/chewing
- It is never too late to stop
- Help is available when you decide to stop

Patient questions
- What withdrawal symptoms might I expect after giving up smoking? How long will they last?
- Are there any withdrawal symptoms particularly associated with my mouth?
- Will I gain weight?
- I smoke low tar cigarettes, so do I need to stop?
- Should I tell people I am trying to stop?
- What should I do when I get an urge to start again?

Assist

- For smokers/chewers wanting to stop appropriate support should be offered
- Do not nag!
- If 'regular' smoker/chewer is interested in quitting, suggest referral to specialist advisers
- Give details of telephone support lines/local advisers
- Consider purchase of NRT gum for low dependency

Arrange

- Monitoring, follow up as appropriate
- 1-2 weeks later check progress
- Support and encouragement

A Practice Protocol for Dealing with Smokers

1. Patient enters practice
2. Information confirmed or sought on smoking status and nicotine dependency
3. Establish interest in quitting
4. Advise all not to smoke
5. If 'irregular light' smoker and interested in quitting, suggest purchase of NRT gum
6. If 'regular' smoker and interested in quitting, suggest referral to specialist advisers
7. Patient record entry
8. Follow up

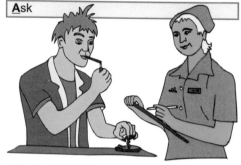

Ask

All patients should have their smoking status checked

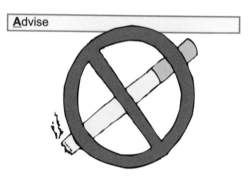

Advise

All smokers should be advised of the value of quitting

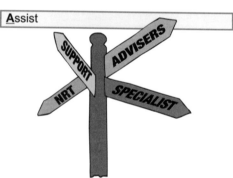

Assist

For those wanting to stop, offer appropriate support

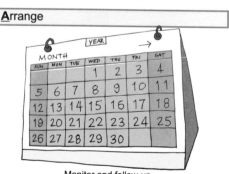

Arrange

Monitor and follow-up

 Remember: The **4A's** for practical approaches to smoking cessation

QUESTIONS

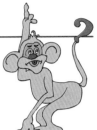

Short Answer Questions

1. Briefly describe four factors that form the basis of a preventive strategy. (2 marks)
2. Briefly describe two types of strategy. (2 marks)
3. What do you understand by the term 'screening'? (1 mark)
4. There are six major fluoride vehicles. Two of these are fluoridated salt and fluoridated mouth rinses. List the remaining four. (2 marks)
5. List one advantage and one disadvantage of using each of them. (2 marks)
6. Name the two risk factors for oral cancer. (1 mark)
7. What is the UK rate of transformation to cancer of (i) leukoplakia and (ii) lichen planus? (1 mark)
8. How does the prevalence of cancers sited on the tongue vary by gender? (1 mark)

Long Answer Questions

Write short notes on the following topics. Up to 4 marks will be awarded for your answer.
1. The principles of screening and their application to periodontal disease.
2. The advantages and disadvantages of water fluoridation over fluoride tablets.
3. The differing approaches that can be adopted to tackle health problems and the role of screening in each of them.
4. Types of strategy to prevent oral disease.
5. The strategies that can be adopted to prevent a health problem.
6. The most appropriate preventive strategies for dental caries among UK children.

Essay Questions

You will be awarded up to 20 marks for your answer.
1. Describe the types of information a consultant in dental public health would collect when conducting a local oral health needs assessment. Outline a range of methods that could be employed to collect this information.
2. List and describe with examples the range of activities you would find within a health promotion strategy. Use this range of activities to develop the content of a health promotion programme to prevent oral cancer.
3. Describe the main barriers to the uptake of dental care. What policy proposals would you make to reduce these barriers? Give reasons for your choice of proposals.

MY NOTES AND SPIDERGRAM

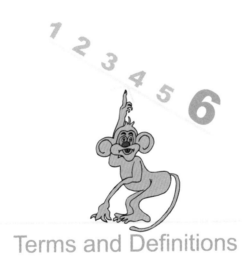

Terms and Definitions

CHAPTER 6

TERMS AND DEFINITIONS (1)

Acceptability
The relationship of clients' attitudes about personal/practice characteristics of providers to the actual characteristics of existing providers.

Access
Is concerned with the ease of availability/accessibility of services as and when they are required.

Accessibility
The relationship between the location of supply and location of clients.

Accommodation
The manner in which supply is organised related to clients' ability to accommodate to these factors (the way care is provided).

Affordability
The relationship of the prices to the clients' income.

Aim
A broad general statement of what you want to achieve.

Availability
The relationship of the volume and type of services to client volume and needs.

Caries
Is a dynamic process involving the exchange of calcium and phosphate ions between tooth structure and saliva (plaque fluid), in the presence of acids produced by the fermentation of carbohydrate by oral microorganisms.

Clinical Governance
A framework designed to improve the quality of health care by identifying ways of improving quality, recognising and managing risk and ensuring continuous professional development.

Common Risk Factor Approach (CRFA)
Maximises resources by targeting risk factors common to many chronic conditions, as many risk factors are related to more than one condition.

Compliance
The degree of constancy and accuracy with which a patient follows a prescribed regimen.

Dental Public Health (DPH)
The science and art of preventing oral disease, promoting oral health and improving the quality of life through the organised efforts of society (Downer *et al.*, 1994).

Disease
Medico-dental defined abnormalities in anatomical structures or physiological or biochemical process.
- *Frequency of disease:* Quantification of the occurrence of disease.
- *Distribution of disease:* Who is getting the disease within a population, where and when the disease is occurring. This includes comparisons of different populations, different sub-groups of same populations, and different periods of observation.
- *Determinants of disease:* What factors are associated with the observed frequency and distribution of disease and how these associations can be tested.

Disease Prevention
Covers measures not only to prevent the occurrence of disease, such as risk factor reduction, but also to arrest its progress and reduce its consequences once established (WHO, 1984).
- *Primary prevention:* Is directed towards preventing the initial occurrence of a disorder.
- *Secondary and tertiary prevention:* Seeks to arrest or retard existing disease and its effects through early detection and appropriate treatment; or to reduce the occurrence of relapses and the establishment of chronic conditions through, for example, effective rehabilitation.

DMF Index
Decay, missing, filled index is the most commonly used method of recording dental caries.

Effectiveness
Is a measure of actual outcome compared to the desired outcome.

Efficiency
Efficiency is a measure of the ratio of actual output to given input.

TERMS AND DEFINITIONS (2)

Epidemiology
The study of the distribution of disease or physiological condition in human populations and of the factors affecting their distribution.
- *Descriptive epidemiology:* Is concerned with the distribution of disease, including consideration of which populations or subgroups do or do not develop a disease, in what geographic location a disease is most or least common, and how the frequency of occurrence varies over time.
- *Analytical epidemiology:* Focuses on the determinants of disease with the ultimate goal of judging whether a particular exposure causes or prevents a specific disease.

Equity
Equity means fairness. The extent to which all individuals in a population can access the care they need (Campbell *et al.,* 2000). Equity can be classified as:
- *Horizontal equity:* Equally accessible effective care for all users, so that persons with equal need receive the same level of health care.
- *Vertical equity:* Greater access to effective care for those with more need, so that greater need for services is met by greater use.

Evaluation
The determination of the effectiveness, efficiency and acceptability of a planned intervention in achieving stated objectives.
- *Outcome evaluation:* What an activity has achieved.
- *Process evaluation:* Explaining how the outcome has been achieved.

Health
The concepts of health are perceived differently by individuals.
- *Health professionals:* Freedom from a medico-dental defined disease.
- *World Health Organization:* A state of complete physical, mental and social well-being and not merely absence of disease (WHO, 1947).

Health Behaviour
Any activity undertaken by an individual, regardless of actual or perceived health status, for the purpose of promoting, protecting or maintaining health, whether or not such behaviour is objectively effective towards that end (Nutbeam, 1998).

Health Care
The health care systems and actions taken within them designed to improve health and well-being (Campbell *et al.,* 2000).

Health Care State
That part of any state concerned with regulating access to, financing and organising the delivery of health care to the population (Moran, 1991).

Health Determinants
The range of personal, social, economic and environmental factors which determine the health status of individuals or populations (Nutbeam, 1998).

Health Education
Is centred around creating opportunities for learning, specifically aimed at producing a health related goal (WHO, 1984).

Health Policy
A consensus on the ideas forming the basis for coordinated plans for action, which in turn ensure that services are provided equitably and healthy environments are maintained (Sheiham, 1996).

Health Promotion
The process of enabling individuals and communities to increase control over the determinants of their health and thereby improve their health (WHO, 1984).

Health System
Comprises all the organisations and resources that are devoted to producing health action and includes all the activities whose primary purpose is to promote, restore and maintain health (WHO, 2000).

TERMS AND DEFINITIONS (3)

Health Work
Carried out by two groups:
- *Formal health work:* That provided by health care professionals, who have undergone specialist training and are paid for their work (e.g. the primary dental care team).
- *Informal health work:* Those people contributing to the maintenance of health and providing care during illness (e.g. self-care, family care, community self-help groups).

Life Long Learning (LLL)
A compulsory re-certification programme in some countries being implemented to promote continuous professional development (CPD). In the UK it consists of 250 hours over a period of 5 years, of which 75 hours must be spent undertaking verifiable CPD. The remainder can be general CPD.

Lifestyle
A way of living based on identifiable patterns of behaviour which are determined by the interplay between an individual's personal characteristics, social interactions, and socio-economic and environmental living conditions.

Locus of Control
Describes perceived control over outcomes (Wallston *et al.,* 1978). There are three classifications:
- *Internal:* A belief that personal action can lead to health outcomes.
- *External/Chance:* Health outcomes are largely controlled by fate.
- *Powerful Others:* Behaviour is in the hands of others, such as dentists.

Negative Predictive Value
The proportion of people with negative test results being correctly labelled non-diseased.

Objective
A specific statement of what you want to achieve within a specific time period.

Oral Health
A standard of health of the oral and related tissues which enables an individual to eat, speak or socialise without active disease, discomfort or embarrassment and which contributes to general well-being.

Periodontal Disease
The term consists of two main broad categories, gingivitis and periodontitis:
- *Gingivitis:* Is an inflammatory response of the gingivae without destruction of the gingivae or their supporting tissues.
- *Periodontitis:* Describes a group of inflammatory diseases affecting all the periodontal structures. It results in destruction of the attachment apparatus and development of a periodontal pocket.

Positive Predictive Value
The proportion of people with positive test results being correctly labelled diseased.

Primary Health Care
Is essential health care made accessible at a cost a country and community can afford, with methods that are practical, scientifically sound and socially acceptable (WHO, 1978).

Quality of Life
An individual's perceptions of their position in life in the context of the culture and value system where they live, and in relation to their goals, expectations, standards and concerns. It is a broad ranging concept, incorporating in a complex way a person's physical health, psychological state, level of independence, social relationships, personal beliefs and relationship to salient features of the environment (WHO, 1996).

Risk Behaviour
Specific forms of behaviour which are proven to be associated with increased susceptibility to a specific disease or ill-health.

Risk Factor
Social, economic or biological status, behaviours or environments which are associated with or cause increased susceptibility to a specific disease, ill-health, or injury.

Screening
Is the presumptive identification of unrecognised disease or defect by the application of tests, examinations or other procedures, which can be applied rapidly (Commission on Chronic Illness, 1957). There are two main types of screening available:
- *Mass screening:* Involves screening on a large scale as the name suggests, e.g. screening the whole population where no selection of population groups is made.
- *Selective screening:* Is aimed specifically at screening high-risk groups.

TERMS AND DEFINITIONS (4)

Self-Efficacy
Belief in one's own ability to bring about a behaviour change effectively (Bandura, 1977).

Sensitivity
The ability of a test to give a positive finding when the person tested truly has the disease.

Specificity
The ability of a test to give a negative finding when the person tested is free of the disease under study.

Strategy
A broad plan of action which specifies what is to be achieved and how to achieve it, and which provides a framework for more detailed planning.

Studies
The different types of study are described below:

- *Longitudinal and Cross-sectional Studies:* Longitudinal studies are those which investigate changes over time (i.e. individuals are observed more than once), whereas cross-sectional studies consist of assessing the status of a group of individuals with respect to the presence or absence of both exposure and disease at the same point in time (i.e. like a snapshot in time).
- *Prospective and Retrospective Studies:* Prospective studies are those in which data are collected forwards in time from the start of the study, whereas retrospective studies are those in which data refer to past events and may be acquired from existing sources.
- *Observational and Interventional Studies:* Observational studies are those in which the researcher collects information on the attributes or measurements of interest, but does not influence events, whereas interventional studies are those in which the researcher deliberately influences events and investigates the effects of the intervention.

Subjective Oral Health Indicators (SOHI)
Measures the extent to which dental and oral disorders disrupt normal social-role functioning and bring about major changes in behaviour.

Trauma
An injury that occurs suddenly and unexpectedly.

MY TERMS AND DEFINITIONS

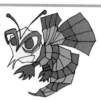

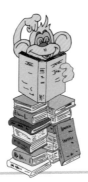

Passing the Exams

THE BRAIN EXPLAINED (1)

Introduction

Weighing in at three pounds (1.4 kilograms) the human brain is quite simply the greatest super computer ever created. The jelly-like mass is thought to have around 10 billion neurons and many more connections between them controlling our thoughts and intelligence. It allows us to think, learn, and to have memories and feelings.

Often students limit their mental capabilities saying things such as 'I can't learn any more'. This is simply not true, as much of our brain is underused. The reasons for statements such as these are usually due to poor time-management, lack of motivation and not understanding the learning process.

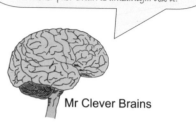

Aoccdrnig to a rscheearch at an Elingsh uinervtisy, it deosn't mttaer in waht oredr the ltteers in a wrod are, the olny iprmoetnt tihng is taht frist and lsat ltteer is at the rghit pclae. The rset can be a toatl mses and you can sitll raed it wouthit porbelm. Tihs is bcuseae we do not raed ervey lteter by itslef but the wrod as a wlohe. Yuor Brian is amzanig... Use it!

Mr Clever Brains

The Stages Of Memory

Immediate Memory hold information for a few seconds or passes it on to your...
Short Term Memory or **Working Memory** holds around seven items of information at once. If the information is not rehearsed immediately, or seen in your head, it will be forgotten in half a minute. The brain filters, discards or chooses information to go on to your...
Long Term Memory is the storage system and retains millions of pieces of data for life. There are several types of memory including visual, auditory and motor memory.

We have five senses, which are our learning channels. We recall events by smell, touch, taste, sound and vision. Some people prefer visual channels of learning as they have strong connections to their visual memory; others prefer the hearing (auditory) channel as they have strong connections to their auditory memory and so on. The best way to learn, however, is through a multi-channel approach by using as many channels as possible, thus giving you the best chance of recalling information.

Sound

Smell

Vision

WE HAVE 5 SENSES WHICH ARE LEARNING CHANNELS

Touch

Taste

Balancing Your Attention Span

1. Keep revision slots between 30 and 40 minutes long with short breaks in-between. This will maintain your attention and concentration, allowing you to learn and hence remember.

2. During your break try to get some fresh air and do something relaxing and unrelated to your work.

3. Avoid things which will inevitably encourage longer breaks, such as calling a friend whom you have not spoken to for a long time or watching the start of your favourite soap...

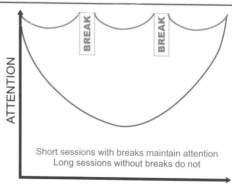

ATTENTION

BREAK

BREAK

TIME

Short sessions with breaks maintain attention
Long sessions without breaks do not

THE BRAIN EXPLAINED (2)

Reviewing

When learning new information, only one fifth of what was understood is remembered after 24 hours. There is an exponential decay of learnt information. Reviewing counteracts the process. Ideally, reviewing the material which may have taken an hour the first time, should take 10-15 minutes the second time and should be done within 24 hours. A third review would take 5-10 minutes and should be done within 72 hours. Review again at the end of the week, which would take several minutes and maintain recall nearer to the 100% recall line. The only difficulty with reviewing is that it requires considerable determination and organisation.

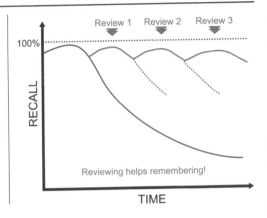

Anxiety And Stress

Anxiety is a normal response to stress. Everyone feels anxious occasionally especially nearing exams. Feelings of panic and loss of control may lead to increasing disorganisation and further panic…leading to a vicious cycle of stress.

It can lead you to avoid the tasks that need to be done. It can also lead to negative thoughts such as 'I'm terrible at exams' or 'I don't know anything'. Although you may feel alone all the other students on your course are in a similar position.

**The important thing is not to panic.
Don't give up…be positive.**

Anxiety is needed to some extent for adequate performance. With increasing levels of anxiety, performance efficiency increases up to an optimum point. Thereafter, additional anxiety leads to lower performance. The key is to achieve the optimal level of anxiety.

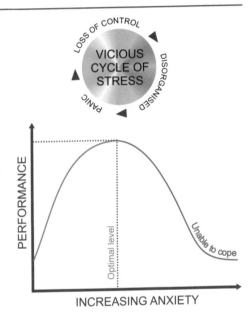

Coping Response

If you feel yourself becoming tense then try to employ breathing and relaxation exercises before and after your revision sessions. You can also de-stress by watching television, playing sports, listening to music or carrying out your favourite hobby. Exercising encourages blood circulation and can also help with keeping you both physically and mentally healthy. Sleeping for around seven to eight hours a night and eating a balanced, healthy diet will help too. Make sure you are well hydrated (not with alcohol though!) and avoid drinking caffeine-rich drinks late in the evening.

If you do feel that the stress is just too much and it is affecting your health, talk about your concerns to a friend, parent, teacher or even a doctor. Talking about your anxieties is a positive step towards dealing with them. It is important to remember that after all, it is only an exam. Keep everything in perspective!

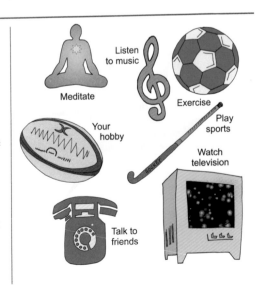

EFFECTIVE REVISION (1)

What Is Revision?

Revision is to re-study something you have already covered by reviewing notes, textbooks and course material in order to understand and remember what you have learnt. Revision requires accurate notes and careful planning.

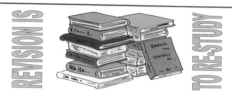

When Do I Start?

There is no correct answer. Some students will have been doing some work throughout the course. Do not be fooled by 'friends' who say they only revise the night before exams! This is either simply not true, or alternatively (and less likely) they are not lying but are more likely to fail. All exams require an element of luck to pass, however, the more work you put in the less luck you need. The bottom line is start in good time. If part-time jobs and social commitments are interfering with your revision, you may need to weigh up the relative benefits of each.

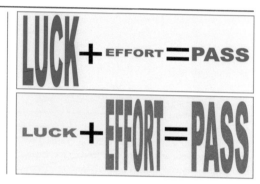

How To Get Started?

Understand the methods of assessment as this will determine what and how you revise. Gain a copy of the syllabus and learning objectives. The syllabus will guide you to areas of weakness that require more attention and those that you know well.

If 5% of your marks are from course work, and the remaining 95% of the marks are from your written papers, you can decide to spend relatively less time on the course work. Find out when, where and what is required for your exam and jot it on your revision calendar, as you do not want to find that you have not got this information the night before the exam.

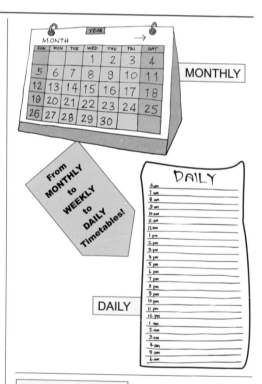

How Long Do I Have?

Most people find that they never have enough time. The important thing here is to make good use of the remaining time and not to panic or give up. Devise a revision timetable of days, weeks (and months) leading up to exams. Fill in the timetable giving a balance of difficult/unfavourable and easy/preferred/interesting subject matter to keep you motivated. Start with the more challenging subject areas so that you know that there are easier ones to follow. If you find yourself getting down, tackle easier topics. In addition to revision-slots, timetable in reward-slots, as these will encourage you to keep on track.

Set realistic targets and leave yourself extra free-slots every so often to catch up on missed topics. When catching up and re-scheduling slots, ask yourself why you did not keep to the timetable… Be truthful to yourself.

There is enough time for both work and play if you have planned properly. Much time is 'wasted', for example, the odd half an hour between lectures, before dinner or between TV programmes that is filled with idle chat or television etc. Over a week, half an hour each day amounts to two and a half hours work. This could leave an evening free to go out with friends.

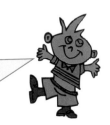

EFFECTIVE REVISION (2)

What Do I Really Need To Know?

Re-examine your syllabus and make a list of major subject areas that need to be covered. Review past papers, which may indicate topics that are frequently examined. This should be an effective guide for your revision. Remember though this does not mean that you miss large chunks of your syllabus. It is important to cover most (if not all) topics to some degree. Identifying topics that you feel unhappy about will allow you to spend more time on these. Remember, you do not need to give all topics equal importance.

Your revision will differ for different assessment methods. Essay questions will require possible essay plans, whereas this would not be true for multiple-choice questions or extended-matching questions.

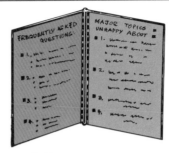

Re-examine
>   **Review**
>   **Revise**
>   **Remember**

Where Do I Revise?

You need to work out where you revise best, be it the library or the kitchen dining table. Some people prefer to work in one place that they associate with study. Others prefer varying their revision location, studying one topic in one place (and then having a break) and studying another topic somewhere else. The following factors influence the effectiveness of your revision:

- **Location:** Choose a quiet, ventilated area where you are unlikely to be disturbed
- **Lighting:** Ensure that there is good lighting
- **Temperature:** Ensure that it is not too cold or warm (which may make you sleepy)
- **Access:** Have all the material in close reach so time is not wasted looking for your textbooks, calculator, pens, papers, notes...
- **Comfort:** Use a comfortable chair and a spacious table/desk
- **Distractions:** Switch off the television and perhaps your phone
- **Music:** Some people find listening to music beneficial, especially calm classical music. Avoid listening to music that is likely to distract you (e.g. encourages you to sing and dance along to it, leave this for the break between the study sessions!)

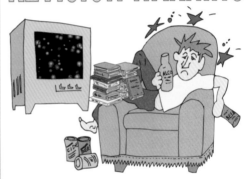

Where Does All My Time Go?

Work out where your time is spent on a daily basis so that you can rearrange your day and make use of any 'wasted' time. Each week you have 168 hours.

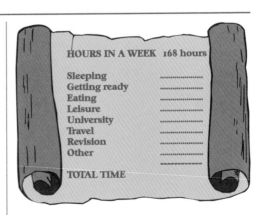

HOURS IN A WEEK 168 hours

Sleeping ....
Getting ready ....
Eating ....
Leisure ....
University ....
Travel ....
Revision ....
Other ....

TOTAL TIME

REVISION AND EXAMINATION TIPS

Revision Tips

'Efficiency is intelligent laziness'   David Dunham

Revision is time-consuming. Make the most of your time spent with the books by using the revision tips below and make your revision efficient!

Mnemonics: The word is derived from the Greek goddess of memory. It is a way of helping you remember information using abbreviations, words or phrases. The funnier, more bizarre or ruder a mnemonic, the more likely you are to remember it. There are many mnemonics and acronyms in this book that will help you remember the key facts that are often tested in exams.

Mind Maps © and Spidergrams: Mind maps have been around for decades and were popularised in the 1960s by Tony Buzan. The graphical nature of these maps helps unlock the potential of the brain. Additionally, the use of many modalities… words, images, numbers, rhythm, colour and spatial awareness… exploits the full range of cortical skills in a solitary powerful approach. These maps are most useful in reviewing topics and for essay plans. Spidergrams are most useful when you have made them yourself. A spidergram of the first chapter has been draw as an example on the next page.

Visual and Auditory Aids: 'Pictures are worth a thousand words'. Make the most of the different parts of your memory by employing pictures and colours. Use diagrams in your answers as they may include additional information that a written answer may miss. Record important information onto an audio format so that you can listen to it whilst in the gym, walking to work etc. The facts are more likely to sink in. You can also try reading out loud, which is another way your brain will register what you are reading.

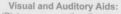
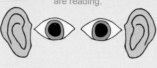

Groups: Working in groups can be more fun and will add variety to your revision. Nevertheless, you must make sure that when you are working in groups, you are actually revising and not just having fun. Remember that if you can teach someone else about a topic, you can be assured that you know the topic well.

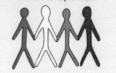

Testing: Remember to try out exam questions, as this will enable you to see which areas require more work.

Notes: Making notes is a form of revising. However, it is important to keep your note-making an active process. This can be done by understanding the material and condensing it into your own words and not by simply copying it out. Some people like to use post-it® notes and stick them around the house or even in textbooks. Do not have too many points on each post-it® as this may confuse you later. Others prefer to have more detailed notes that they will then summarise and later further summarise. Highlighting in different colours may also help you remember.

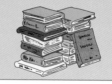

'If we did the things we are capable of, we would astound ourselves'   Thomas Edison

Examination Tips

Before the Exam

- Make sure you know where and when your exams are to be held.
- Make sure you have the right equipment (i.e. calculators, student ID cards, pens) for each exam.
- Dress appropriately in comfortable clothing (e.g. an oral viva may require smart clothes).
- Go to the toilet before the exam.

During the Exam

- Read the instructions very carefully so that you know how many questions you have to answer, whether any questions are compulsory and how long you have.
- Time the exam so that you spend the right amount of time answering each question. If you only attempt half the paper, the maximum you can score is 50% (and it is unlikely that you will get all the marks!).
- Read the questions very carefully before you put pen to paper and not halfway through your answer. Underline key words in the question. If it is an essay, then spend some time planning it so that you avoid jumbling your ideas.
- Answer what is asked of you, not what you hope they are asking. No matter how good your work is, if you do not answer the question, you will not get the marks.
- Make sure your answers are clearly presented, if the examiner cannot read them, they cannot give you the marks. Write legibly and label your diagrams.
- Leave time at the end to check for mistakes.

After the Exam

- Do not get worked up about the exam you have just taken, you cannot do anything about it now! Focus on the next exam if there is one. If not, go and party!
- If your performance was affected by sickness or another situation, tell your tutor without delay (preferably before the exam).

'Obstacles are things a person sees when he takes his eyes off his goal'   E. Joseph Cossman

Exams are a part of life. Although they do not count for everything, they can lead to new opportunities. Face them with a positive attitude and you are likely to succeed… Good luck!

SPIDERGRAM OF CHAPTER 1

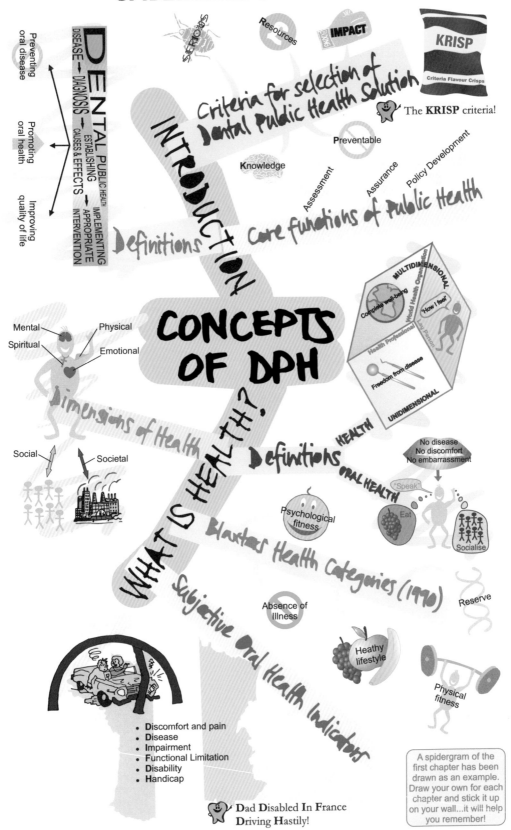

Serious

Resources

IMPACT

KRISP
Criteria Flavour Crisps

Criteria for selection of Dental Public Health solution

The **KRISP** criteria!

Preventable

Knowledge

DENTAL PUBLIC HEALTH
DISEASE → DIAGNOSIS → ESTABLISHING CAUSES & EFFECTS → IMPLEMENTING APPROPRIATE INTERVENTION

Preventing oral disease

Promoting oral health

Improving quality of life

INTRODUCTION

Definitions

Core functions of Public Health

Assessment   Assurance   Policy Development

CONCEPTS OF DPH

MULTIDIMENSIONAL
World Health Organisation
Complete well-being
'How I feel'
Health Professional   Lay Person
Freedom from disease
UNIDIMENSIONAL

Mental   Physical
Spiritual   Emotional

Dimensions of Health

Social   Societal

Definitions   HEALTH
ORAL HEALTH

No disease
No discomfort
No embarrassment

"Speak"

Eat

Socialise

WHAT IS HEALTH?

Psychological fitness

Blaxter's Health Categories (1990)

Reserve

Subjective Oral Health Indicators

Absence of Illness

Heathy lifestyle

Physical fitness

- Discomfort and pain
- Disease
- Impairment
- Functional Limitation
- Disability
- Handicap

Dad **D**isabled **I**n **F**rance **D**riving **H**astily!

A spidergram of the first chapter has been drawn as an example. Draw your own for each chapter and stick it up on your wall...it will help you remember!

REFERENCES (1)

Acheson D. (1998). *Independent Inquiry into Health Inequalities in Health: a report.* London, The Stationery Office.

Anderson RJ and Morgan JD. (1992). Marketing dentistry: a pilot study in Dudley. *Community Dental Health.* 9 Suppl 1:1-220.

Andreasen J and Andreasen E. (1994). *Textbook and Colour Atlas of Traumatic Injuries to Teeth.* Copenhagen, Munksgaard.

Bandura A. (1977). Self-efficacy: toward a unifying theory of behavioral change. *Psychological Review.* 84:191-215.

Bandura A. (1977). *Social Learning Theory.* London, Prentice Hall.

Bauer JC, Pierson AP and House DR. (1978). *Factors Which Affect the Utilization of Dental Services, a Review and Analysis of the Literature.* DHEW Publication No. (HRA) 78-64. Hyattsville, Maryland, US Department of Health, Education and Welfare.

Blaxter M. (1990). *Health and Lifestyles.* London, Tavistock.

Chestnutt IG. (1998). Chapter 1: Psychological aspects of dental care. In: Chestnutt IG, Gibson J. *Churchill's Pocketbook of Clinical Dentistry.* Singapore, Churchill Livingstone.

Dahlgren G and Whitehead M. (1993). *Tackling Social Inequalities in Health: what can we learn from what has been tried?* Technical Background Paper for International Seminar on Tackling Inequalities in Health. Ditchley Park, Oxford. London, King's Fund.

Donabedian A. (1974). *Aspects of Medical Care Administration: specifying requirements for health care.* Cambridge, Massachusetts, Harvard University Press.

Donabedian A. (1990). The seven pillars of quality. *Archives of Pathology and Laboratory Medicine.* 114:1115-1118.

Downer MC, Gelbier S and Gibbons DE. (1994). *Introduction to Dental Public Health.* London, FDI World Press.

Dubos R. (1979). *Mirage of Health.* New York, Harper Colophan.

Ewles L and Simnett I. (1999). *Promoting Health: a practical guide to health education.* London, Baillière-Tindall.

Finch H, Keegar J, Ward K and Sanyal Sen B. (1988). *Barriers to the Receipt of Dental Care.* London, British Dental Association.

General Dental Council. (2000). *The First Five Years.* London, General Dental Council.

Gift HC, Andersen RM and Chen M. (1997). Chapter 16: The principles of organization and models of delivery of oral health care. In: Pine CM. *Community Oral Health.* Oxford, Wright.

Glass RL. (1982). The first international conference on the declining prevalence of dental caries. The evidence and the impact on dental education, dental research and dental practice. *Journal of Dental Research.* 61:1301-1383.

Glendor U, Marcenes W and Andreasen JO. (2006). Chapter 3: Classification, epidemiology and etiology. In: *Textbook and Color Atlas of Traumatic Dental Injuries to the Teeth* (4th edition). In press.

Golder M. (1995). Non-accidental injury in children. *Dental Update.* 22:75-80.

Goodson J, Tamer A, Haffajee A *et al.* (1982). Patterns of progression and digression of advanced destructive periodontal disease. *Journal of Clinical Periodontology.* 9:472-481.

Gratrix D and Holloway PJ. (1994). Factors of deprivation associated with dental caries in young children. *Community Dental Health.* 11:66-70.

Gray PG, Todd JE, Slack GL and Bulman JS. (1970). *Government Social Survey: adult dental health in England and Wales in 1968.* London, HMSO.

Green LW and Kreuter MW. (1991). *Health Promotion Planning: an educational and environmental approach.* California, Mayfield.

Hobdell M, Petersen PE, Clarkson J and Johnson N. Global goals for oral health 2020. *International Dental Journal.* 53:285-288.

Illich I. (1976). *Medical Nemesis: the expropriation of health.* New York, Bantam Books.

Jacob C and Plamping D. (1989). *The Practice of Primary Dental Care.* London, Wright.

Kelly M, Steele J, Nuttal N, Bradnock G, Morris J, Nunn J, Pine C, Pitts N, Treasure E and White D. (2000). *Adult Dental Health Survey: oral health in the United Kingdom 1998.* London, The Stationery Office.

Kidd EAM and Joyston-Bechal S. (1987). *Essentials of Dental Caries* (second edition). Hong Kong, Oxford University Press.

Lalonde M. (1974). *A New Perspective on the Health of Canadians: a working document.* Ottawa, Health and Welfare Canada.

Levine R. (2001). *The Scientific Basis of Dental Health Education: a policy document* (fourth edition). London, Health Development Agency.

Locker D. (1988). Measuring oral health: a conceptual framework. *Community Dental Health.* 5:3-18.

Longmore M, Wilkinson IB and Rajagopalan S. (2004). *Oxford Handbook of Clinical Medicine* (sixth edition). Oxford, Oxford University Press.

Marcenes W, Freysleben GR and Peres MA. Contribution of changing diagnostic criteria toward reduction of caries between 1971 and 1997 in children attending the same school in Florianopolis, Brazil. *Community Dentistry and Oral Epidemiology.* 29:449-455.

Maxwell RJ. (1984). Quality assessment in health. *British Medical Journal (Clinical Research Edition).* 228:1470-1472.

McKeown T. (1979). *The Role of Medicine.* Oxford, Basil Blackwell.

Nadanovsky P and Sheiham A. Relative contribution of dental services to the changes in caries levels of 12-year-old children in 18 industrialized countries in the 1970s and early 1980s. *Community Dentistry and Oral Epidemiology.* 23:331-339.

Newton JT, Corrigan M, Gibbons DE and Locker D. (2003). The self-assessed oral health status of individuals from White, Indian, Chinese and Black Caribbean communities in South-east England. *Community Dentistry and Oral Epidemiology.* 31:192-199.

Nutbeam D. (1998). *World Health Organization: health promotion glossary.* Switzerland, World Health Organization.

Office of National Statistics. (2003). *Children's Dental Health 2003: preliminary findings.* London Office for National Statistics. [http://www.statistics.gov.uk/]

Office for National Statistics. (2004). *Cancer Statistics Registrations: registrations of cancer diagnosed in 2001, England.* Series MB1. London Office for National Statistics. [http://www.statistics.gov.uk/]

Office for National Statistics. (2004). *Mortality Statistics: cause, England and Wales.* Series DH2. London Office for National Statistics. [http://www.statistics.gov.uk/]

Papapanou PN. (1996). Periodontal diseases: epidemiology. *Annals of Periodontology.* 1:1-36.

Penchansky R and Thomas JW. (1981). The concept of access: definition and relationship to consumer satisfaction. *Medical Care.* 19:127-140.

Pitts N and Harker R. (2003). *Obvious Decay Experience: children's dental health in the United Kingdom 2003.* London, Office for National Statistics.

Prochaska JO and DiClemente CC. (1983). Stages and processes of self-change of smoking: toward an integrative model of change. *Journal of Consulting and Clinical Psychology.* 51:390-395.

Sheiham A. (1984). Changing trends in dental caries. *International Journal of Epidemiology.* 13:142-147.

Sheiham A. (1991). Why free sugars consumption should be below 15 kg per person per year in industrialised countries: the dental evidence. *British Dental Journal.* 171:63-65.

Sheiham A. (1997). Impact of dental treatment on the incidence of dental caries in children and adults. *Community Dentistry and Oral Epidemiology.* 25:104-112.

Sheiham A and Watt RG. (2000). The common risk factor approach: a rational basis for promoting oral health. *Community Dentistry and Oral Epidemiology.* 28:399-406.

Socransky S, Haffajee A, Goodson J and Linde J. (1984). New concepts of destructive periodontal disease. *Journal of Clinical Periodontology.* 11:21-32.

Townsend P, Davidson N and Whitehead M. (1992). *Inequalities in Health: the Black Report and the health divide.* London, Penguin.

Turnock BJ, Handler A, Hall W, Potsic S, Nalluri R and Vaughn EH. (1994). Local health department effectiveness in addressing the core functions of public health. *Journal of the US Public Health Service.* 109:653-658.

Walker A and Cooper I. (1998). *Adult Dental Health Survey: Oral Health in the United Kingdom 1998.* London, Office for National Statistics.

REFERENCES (3)

Wallston KA, Wallston BS and DeVellis R. (1978). Development of the multidimensional health locus of control (MHLC) scales. *Health Education Monographs.* 6:160-170.

Watt RG. (1997). Stages of change for sugar and fat reduction in an adolescent sample. *Community Dental Health.* 14:102-107.

Watt RG, Daly B and Kay EJ. (2003). Prevention. Part 1: smoking cessation advice within the general dental practice. *British Dental Journal.* 194:665-668.

Wiebe CB and Putnins EE. The periodontal disease classification system of the American Academy of Periodontology: an update. *Journal of the Canadian Dental Association.* 66:594-597.

WHO. (1984). *Health Promotion: a discussion document on the concepts and principles.* Copenhagen, World Health Organization.

WHO. (1986). *The Ottawa Charter for Health Promotion.* Geneva, World Health Organization.

WHO. (1986). *The Health Promotion Logo.* Geneva, World Health Organization.

WEBSITES

British Dental Association (BDA) www.bda-dentistry.org.uk
The professional association and trade union for dentists in the UK

British Dental Health Foundation (BDHF) www.dentalhealth.org.uk
The BDHF is a charity dedicated to raising public awareness of dental and oral health and promoting good dental health practices

British Fluoridation Society (BFS) www.bfsweb.org
Provides evidence-based information on fluoride and all aspects of water fluoridation

Centre for Evidence-based Dentistry www.cebd.org
An independent body whose aim is to promote the teaching, learning, practice and evaluation of evidence-based dentistry world-wide

Centre for Reviews and Dissemination www.york.ac.uk/inst/crd
Information on how to undertake systematic reviews, together with databases of review appraisals

Dental Vocational Training Authority (DVTA) www.dvta.nhs.uk
Postgraduate organisation for continuing education

Department of Health (DoH) www.dh.gov.uk
Official website of UK Department of Health, the government department responsible for public health issues

General Dental Council (GDC) www.gdc-uk.org
Organisation that regulates dental professionals in the UK

National Statistics www.statistics.gov.uk
Official statistics on the UK's economy, population and society

Royal Society of Medicine (RSM) www.rsm.ac.uk
An independent, apolitical organisation of doctors, dentists, scientists and others involved in medicine and health care

The Cochrane Collaboration www.cochrane.org
International non-profit organisation preparing, maintaining and promoting accessibility of systematic reviews of the effects of health care initiatives

The Public Health electronic Library (PHeL) www.phel.gov.uk
Provides knowledge and know-how to promote health, prevent disease and reduce health inequalities

United Nations (UN) www.un.org
Global association of governments facilitating cooperation in international law, security, economic development and social equity

World Health Organization (WHO) www.who.int
The WHO is the United Nations specialised agency for health

EPIDEMIOLOGICAL DATA

Adult Dental Health Survey National survey every 10 years of adults 16+ years old

Child Dental Health Survey National survey every 10 years of children 5-15 years old

British Association for the Study of Community Dentistry (BASCD) Survey Local survey of 5, 12, 14 year-olds

General Household Survey Multi-purpose continuous survey started in 1971 which collects information on a range of topics from people living in private households in Great Britain

National Census A survey of all people and households in the UK

National Diet and Nutrition Survey (NDNS) A survey of 19-64 year olds of the dietary habits and the nutritional status of the population of Great Britain

Useful website for epidemiological data: National Statistics www.statistics.gov.uk (see above)

BOOKS

Bowling A. (1997). *Research Methods in Health*. Buckingham, Open University Press.

Daly B, Watt RG, Batchelor P and Treasure ET. (2003). *Essential Dental Public Health*. Oxford, Oxford University Press.

Davey B, Gray A and Seale C (eds). (1995). *Health and Disease: a reader* (second edition). Buckingham, Open University Press.

Ewles L and Simnett I. (1998). *Promoting Health: a practical guide to health education* (fourth edition). London, Scutari Press.

Kent GC and Croucher R. (1998). *Achieving Oral Health: the social context of dentistry*. Oxford, Butterworth-Heinemann.

Marmot M and Wilkinson RG. (1999). *Social Determinants of Health*. Oxford, Oxford University Press.

Marshall L and Rowland F. (1998). *A Guide to Learning Independently* (third edition). Buckingham, Open University Press.

Murray JJ, Nunn J and Steele J. (2003). *The Prevention of Oral Disease*. Oxford, Oxford Medical Publications.

Naidoo J and Wills J. (2000). *Health Promotion: foundations for practice*. London, Baillière-Tindall.

Pine CM (ed). (1997). *Community Oral Health*. London, Butterworth-Heinemann.

Rowntree D. (1981). *Statistics Without Tears: a primer for non-mathematicians*. Harmondsworth, Penguin Books.

World Health Organization. (2003). *The World Oral Health Report 2003: Continuous improvement of oral health in the 21st century: the approach of the WHO Global Oral Health Programme*. Geneva, World Health Organization.

NOTES

SPIDERGRAM

NOTES

SPIDERGRAM

NOTES

INDEX